MADWIVES

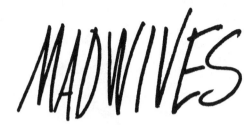

SCHIZOPHRENIC WOMEN IN THE 1950s

CAROL A. B. WARREN

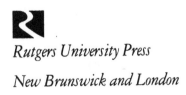

Rutgers University Press

New Brunswick and London

Appendix A is a revised version of the appendix to *Schizophrenic Women: Studies in Marital Crisis,* by Harold Sampson, Sheldon L. Messinger, and Robert D. Towne. Copyright © Lieber-Atherton, Inc., 1964.

Appendix B is a revised version of "Clinical and Research Interviewing in Sociology," by Carol A. B. Warren, *Clinical Sociology Review* 3 (1985): 72–84.

Library of Congress Cataloging-in-Publication Data

Warren, Carol A. B., 1944–
  Madwives : schizophrenic women in the 1950s.

  Bibliography: p.
  Includes index.
    1. Housewives—Mental health—California—
San Francisco Bay Area—History—20th century.
2. Housewives—California—San Francisco Bay Area—Interviews.   3. Schizophrenics—California—
San Francisco Bay Area—Interviews.   4. Schizophrenia—
Treatment—California—History—20th century.
5. Psychiatric hospital care—California—History—
20th century.   6. Sex role—California—History—20th
century. I. Title. [DNLM: 1. Hospitalization.
2. Hospitals, Psychiatric—history—California.
3. Identification (Psychology) 4. Schizophrenia—
history—California.   5. Schizophrenia—in adulthood.
6. Women.   WM 11 AC2   W2m]
RC451.4.H68W37   1987   362.2'088042   86-14620
  ISBN: 978-0-8135-1689-9
British Cataloging-in-Publication information available

For my husband Bill and my son Ian, with love

Contents

Preface

This book is about life as a woman, marriage, and mental hospitalization in the 1950s. It is based on the lives of seventeen women who were diagnosed as schizophrenic, institutionalized in Napa State Hospital in California, and then released. It is also about their husbands, their children, and their social circles. It is, in short, a study of gender.

The interviews on which the study is based—which are called, by those who have worked with them, the "Bay Area data"—were conducted between late 1957 and early 1961 by a team of researchers associated with the University of California: Sheldon L. Messinger, Robert Towne, Harold Sampson, David Ross, Florine Livson, Mary Bowers, Lester Cohen, and Kate Dorst. The original study was designed to examine the impact of mental hospitalization on families over a thirty-six-month period, beginning with the first week of admission and ending as much as a year after discharge.

Case summaries of these women and their families are given in appendix A. I use the pseudonyms invented for the first study (Sampson et al. 1964): the Arlens, Bakers, Jameses, Karrs, Lows, Marks, Noons, Orens, Prices, Quinns, Rands, Sands, Thornes, Ureys, Vicks, Whites, and Yales. Of these families all but the Bakers, Jameses, Lows, Prices, and Quinns were reinterviewed in 1972; these interviews provide the material for the epilogue. In order to protect the respondents' identities, I have changed many details concerning the lives of the Bay Area respondents from both the original and 1972 interviews and Sampson et al. (1964).

I came to this study by chance, as a result of meeting one of the original researchers, Sheldon L. Messinger, at a convention of the Association for Criminal Justice Researchers. I was interested in the mental-health system; he asked me if I would like to look at the interviews with these families. I was indeed interested, and became increasingly so over the years. Following a period of several months in which I commuted to Berkeley from Los Angeles to examine the interviews, Shelly found the only way to get me out of his office and shipped the transcripts to me in Los Angeles. Today these approximately fifteen thousand pages of interviews live (in a purple form that echoes a precomputer, indeed pre-photocopier technology) in four filing-cabinet drawers in my office.

A number of publications between the 1960s and the 1980s have been based directly or indirectly on the Bay Area data, including, of course, the researchers' initial report, entitled *Schizophrenic Women: Studies in Marital Crisis* (Sampson et al. 1964). The purposes of the original study, funded by the National Institute of Mental Health, were stated as follows:

The period we are attempting to describe encompasses a sequence of organization–disorganization–reorganization. We shall trace in some detail the development of the crises which led to the admission of these women to the state mental hospital and the ways in which these crises were modified during hospitalization and following release. Our broad aim is to describe this extended segment of the careers of these women and their marital families and to understand these careers as shaped by and as parts of family and institutional processes. (Sampson et al. 1964, 2)

The original study focused on the psychodynamics of the mother–daughter–husband triad (sometimes including the mother-in-law) as it served to precipitate the crisis of hospitalization. By contrast, the focus of my study is on gender, trouble, and the husband–wife dyad. I am particularly interested in the way that roles in the traditional family structure of the 1950s, together with psychiatric law and practice, caused women's experience of emotional trouble to be perceived as schizophrenic and as requiring mental hospitalization. My point is not that mental hospitalization was not a crisis for these families, nor that psychodynamic processes were irrelevant to the women's schizophrenic episodes. What I would argue is that, from the perspective of the 1980s, the frameworks of gender roles and trouble in the 1950s are particularly revealing: the one because it highlights the stress and inequality in traditional families, and the other because it formulates a perception of troubles in ordinary life as progressing to a sense of crisis.

There are many people without whom this book could not have been written. My very special thanks go to Sheldon Messinger, not only for introducing me to the Bay Area families, but also for his insightful suggestions and comments on this and other manuscripts. I am also grateful to John Clausen, who gave me access to the 1972 follow-up interviews with the families and who provided suggestions for the development of my analysis. I must also, though unfortunately posthumously, acknowledge the role of Erving Goffman in the development of this study, since it was he who first suggested the importance of the housewife role in understanding these women's experiences. In addition, Randall Collins, Richard Levinson, Alan Horwitz, Barbara Laslett, Linda Fuller, and Jennifer Glass, and in particular Robert Emerson, provided useful comments at various stages of the manuscript's development.

Other people were also very helpful in the process. Elaine Corry and Judith Webb first taught me to use the word processor. Several people were invaluable in typing various sections of the manuscript when I proved to be a most umpromising pupil: Jindarat P. Lau, Melinda Welch, Maria Greene, Mary Sears, and Nancy Raman. The Rockefeller Foundation—and in particular Roberto and Gianna Celli and Angela Barmettler—made it possible for me to spend a month at the Villa Serbelloni in Bellagio, Italy, which gave me the time and the facilities to revise several sections of the manuscript.

Finally I want to thank my husband, William G. Staples, for his unfailing support, his fellow-sociologist's intellectual sharing, and his lessons in word processing (which finally took); and my son, Ian Warren Staples, for being born, and for being such a joy. Without their love this book would have been much more difficult to contemplate and to complete.

Introduction

CHAPTER 1

Women, Trouble, and Madness

The purpose of this book is to understand the social and historical processes through which certain wives in the 1950s became madwives. I am particularly interested in the ways in which gender and the dynamics of marital relationships shaped these processes, transforming various sorts of emotional and role troubles into schizophrenia. I approach my task with a particular view of theory and methods, a stance that is sometimes referred to as interpretive. The interpretive approach to social science sees theory and method as part of a hermeneutic process of understanding, a process that is historical, interactional, and individual. As Peter Barham says of social action, its "characterization . . . requires of us that we grapple with the interconnections between the intentional, the social and the historical. . . . So, for example, the history of a particular individual within a particular marriage is set within the history of development of the institution of marriage. An action, or a set of actions, is thus an episode in an individual history that must be viewed in the context of a history of a setting" (1984, 88–89). And, similarly, the history of a particular individual who is "mentally ill" is set within the history of the development of psychiatry.

Interpretive sociology, with its emphasis on the individual, the social, and the historical, is neither positivistic in method, nor hypothesis-testing in theoretical intent. Furthermore, the process of interpretation is one in which the analyst is a fundamental part of the hermeneutic circle. The separation of research into theory, methods, and "objective" analyst is replaced by a sense of the unity of all these elements with the data. Interpretive work is based on a different logic from positivistic work, proposing that "scientific reason is dependent on historical reason" (ibid., 63), and that "the starting point for inquiry is bound to be the dialectical situation in which one finds oneself caught in one's own historical period . . . traditional notions of 'objectivity' and 'scientific method' must be abandoned" (ibid., 75).

The use of an interpretive perspective has a number of implications for the conduct of sociological inquiry. First, the reanalysis of data is defined in a particular way. A positivistic research model would approach re-analysis as an exercise in reliability, the logic of which requires that any subsequent study, including mine, reconfirm the findings of *Schizophrenic Women* (Sampson et al. 1964). But an interpretive framework, with its insistence on historically and biographically grounded understanding, would expect a new analysis to differ from earlier ones. Thus, my analysis is informed by critical commentary in feminist theory, gender roles, and other aspects of a changing intellectual tradition that has altered the face of social inquiry since the 1950s. My analysis neither replicates nor invalidates the original; rather, it differs historically and biographically from it. As Sheldon Messinger commented when he read this book, "in addition to the fact that Sampson et al. employed a different interpretive frame on the completed interviews (the psychodynamic and crisis foci), the interviewees themselves reflected the fact that Sampson et al., like the subjects themselves—if slightly less so—tended to take family gender norms for granted."

The second characteristic of interpretive inquiry is that data, theory, and method are seen not as fundamentally different tasks, but as different aspects of the same process. Theories and methods themselves are seen as historically grounded rather than as ahistorical truths and technologies. The task of this book, then, is neither to test theories (of mental illness or of gender's contribution to it) nor to develop an ethnographically grounded theory of interaction. It is to understand the experience of mental illness in the fifties as an experience of persons, of families, and within history.

Erving Goffman's studies of the moral career of the mental patient (1961; 1971) and Robert Emerson and Sheldon Messinger's analysis of the micropolitics of trouble (1977)—both transformed from un-gendered to gendered models—form the conceptual basis of my discussion of the mental-hospitalization process. Goffman divides the moral career of the mental patient into the prepatient, patient, and ex-patient stages, with their focal concerns of family relations, staff–patient interactions, and stigma (1961). Emerson and Messinger propose that the micro- or interactional politics of trouble are embedded in a "macro-politics," in which "broader economic and social interests shape both the frames of reference and the institutionalized remedies available for identifying and dealing with the trouble" (1977, 132). This study is at the intersection of the macro- and micropolitics of trouble.

What I want to do is to place in contexts both of gender and of history Goffman's theory of the mental patient's moral career, which he elaborates in his classic ethnography of the mental hospital, *Asylums* (1961). Goffman's theory attends explicitly to neither of these contexts, though both are to some degree implicit in the analysis. The experiences of the hospitalized mental patient, as well as the steps leading up to hospitalization and away from it, are profoundly affected by the gender of the several parties to these processes and by many aspects of the historical context. For example, both legal and diagnostic practices at a particular time and place are involved in the decision to commit someone involuntarily to a mental hospital, but so is whether the proposed inpatient is a man or woman.

Space considerations prohibit a full discussion of the original methods of sample selection and data analysis, which can be found in Sampson et al. (1964). Briefly, the Bay Area respondents were selected on a "convenience" basis: every patient who was admitted to Napa State Hospital during the early weeks of the study who also met the sampling criteria was added to the sample. These criteria were: the women were all first admissions (after some considerable work had been done on them, the original researchers found that Ann Rand and Kate White had had earlier, brief psychiatric-hospital admissions), white, married, between the ages of twenty-six and forty, and with at least one child living at home. The bulk of the data collected were in the form of intensive interviews over a period of thirty-six months, with one member of the research team of eight social scientists. Approximately half the interviews were tape-recorded and transcribed.

Intensive interviews of this type are often treated as the "poor cousins" of ethnographic research, at least by the standard qualitative-methods texts (see, for example, Lofland and Lofland 1984). Indeed, the radical perspective on interviews is that they are accounts, not documents: they refer only to the interview moment and the interview relationship, and to no other moments or relationships (Smith 1978; 1983). Obviously, in using interviews to illuminate the place of women in the fifties I do not share this radical critique (see appendix B for a discussion of intensive interviews).

The process of data analysis as I engaged in it is described in standard-methods texts such as Lofland and Lofland (1984). Interpretation of qualitative data consists of repeatedly reading the material in order to develop analytic themes and categories from the intersection of the data with the analyst's own understandings of the world. This process is reflexive, with prior understandings being modified by immersion in new data and the reinterpretation of the data undergoing continuous revision from the original vision, incorporating the views of reviewers and editors as well as of the author. My analysis moves from the larger social context in which these women's troubles occurred to the inner reaches of the self, and through the moral career of the madwife. Part I is concerned mainly with the prepatient, part II with the inpatient, and part III with the female ex-patient in the fifties. I say "mainly" because, in contrast to ethnographic observation, the intensive-interview method highlights processual and overlapping features of biography not easily separable into discrete stages. For example, electroconvulsive therapy (ECT), discussed in chapter 5, was significant in the lives of these families both during and after hospitalization.

The Problem of History

Designating this study of the fifties as "history" has engaged me in a lively debate with reviewers and other colleagues over what that term means. As I see it, there are two issues to be confronted in designating this work as "historical": one is the interpretation of historical change within a capitalist state (a temporal and epistemological problem), and the other is justifying the designation of data as "historical" or "contemporary" (a temporal and disciplinary problem).

Historical studies—especially those taking into account the political economy—refer to a broad period of capitalist or "state" society within which equally broad generalizations obtain: there is a particular sort of division of labor, class relations are based on private property, and families—like all other social relations—are shaped by the overarching metaphor of the marketplace and the long arm of state regulation (this subject is discussed at greater length below). This historical period stretches, very roughly, from the mid-nineteenth century to the present (although one of the features of contemporary historiography is that temporal boundaries are continually being pushed backward). The feminist family sociology of Heidi Hartmann is in this tradition, arguing that there has been little change in traditional gender roles during this "capitalist" era. But other scholars argue that it is necessary to make distinctions between historical epochs much more narrowly conceived, say, the 1950s versus the 1970s. The historical family demography of Andrew Cherlin is based on this concept of epochs, focusing on differences and transition periods between these decades.

Both of these approaches to history are valuable in understanding the fifties. This decade is part of the long process of capitalist-society development, but it is also a transition period, which displays the elaboration of particular historical themes. The fifties were both part of an era and a moment poised between the certainties of post–World War II culture and the disruptions and upheavals of the sixties. In the portrait of marital and family relations revealed by the Bay Area interviews, for example, one can trace the sort of traditional gender-role arrangements still to be found in American society today. But at the same time, one can also find a style of marital commitment—a modern might call it endurance—that is uncommon in the eighties world of relational disenchantment and high divorce rate. Similarly, the post-Vietnam era saw a great re-awakening of feminist consciousness, one taking a number of new forms, which was dormant in the fifties and early sixties (Margolis 1984). Troubled housewives today have a legitimating cultural vocabulary that was virtually absent from the lives of these troubled madwives in the early months of 1958. The Bay Area women were not only isolated in their households—as many, though far fewer, housewives are today—but they were also isolated in their sense of protest against the impera-tives of role.

In addition, the seventies and eighties have seen a transformation, in California and nationwide, in the mental health system through which today's women and men are committed or admit themselves to mental hospitals. The state mental hospitals have been "emptied"—partly rhe-torically and partly in fact—of their long-term inmates. Contemporary wives cannot so easily be transformed, through the collusion of hus-bandly and psychiatric authority, into mental patients. Through a num-ber of economic and legal changes, women are no longer as economically dependent on their husbands or as vulnerable to involuntary psychiatry as they were twenty-five years ago. And yet the cultural association between women and madness is still very strong (Chesler 1972; Schur 1984). While the Bay Area data may be seen in the short term as revealing a society in transition, it must also be seen in the long term as an empirical record of essentially unaltered (though not unalterable) capitalist societal forms.

At the same time, societal conditions over the long term have not changed enough to bring about fundamental alterations in either gender roles or the conditions of mental patients. Women still do far more housework than men; mental patients are still placed in bureaucratic medical organizations, which place a premium on social control and conformity. The great social transformations we refer to as capitalism, industrialization, and bureaucratization have not themselves been transformed; thus the basic societal formations that flow from them may change in detail, but not in principle. As a consequence of this dual view of history, I will indicate, in this chapter, what I see as particular to the fifties and what has been more enduring over time.

The second problem of history can be seen as a problem in the history of social science. To take an example, nobody would insist that a study done in 1853 was contemporary or that one done in 1983 was historical—though these temporal distinctions are in fact arbitrary. But the fifties appear to have no such clear-cut character.

Between the contemporary and the historical, however defined, lies a zone of conventional ambiguity that scholars cannot frame satisfactorily as either. The fifties have been within this zone for a decade or so, virtually untouchable either by history or by the sociology of contemporary life. But this view of the fifties has been changing very recently—though not the temporal conventions it implies. Both I and several historians were asked to give talks on gender relations in the fifties at the 1986 convention of the Organization of American Historians. The official seal of history has been extended to the era.

Thus I hope that this book will be of interest to historians as well as sociologists, to structuralist scholars interested in the way in which gender enters the social process, and to social scientists who specialize in the fifties. I would be pleased if family sociologists and psychiatric sociologists found in it insights useful for the development of their theories, and if interactionists should judge it grounded enough to be worthy of their attention. Although the work is historical, and by no means etiological, it is possible that clinicians and others interested in helping the troubled will derive some useful understanding of the way mental patients interpret the diagnoses and treatments that are extended to them.

In the 1950s, the process of mental illness and hospitalization often occurred within the context of what is referred to as the "traditional family." What was "traditional" was the separated roles of women and men in the household and in the workplace. The role of the typical fifties male centered around his function as economic provider; that of the typical fifties female centered around her functions as housewife and mother. The household role of women depended on the provider role of the husband; the economic situation of men and women was one of control and dependence, respectively. This economic relationship was mirrored in the marital relationship in general (André 1981; Hartmann 1981) and in the psychiatric and legal subordination of women (Margolis 1984; Matthews 1984).

Beyond sharing the social place of married women in the fifties, madwives had behaved in ways, or experienced feelings, that had led themselves or others to regard them as mental patients. We shall see, as their story unfolds, that the pathways to Napa State Hospital of even such a small number of women as seventeen were extremely diverse. They ranged from one woman, Peggy Sand, who wanted to get away from her abusive husband; to another, Mary Yale, who thought she was turning into a man; and another, Donna Urey, who burned down her house. Madwives are not *all* wives, in the fifties or at any other time; but they reflect within their individual experiences the collective experiences of the era.

The traditional marital relationship of the fifties was the context within which the Bay Area women experienced the moral career of the mental patient. All the women were married at the time of the study; five of the wives and two of the husbands had been previously married. Nine of the women had been married to their current husbands from between two and ten years, and eight from eleven to sixteen years. They had between one and five children in the household, with an age range of six months to sixteen years; they were between twenty-six and forty years old with a mean of thirty-five, and they were all white. The median length of stay at Napa for the women (from first admission to first release) was nineteen weeks. The shortest stay was six weeks, and the longest was sixty-four weeks (see table 1.1).

In contemporary society the family (Goffman 1971) and especially

TABLE 1.1

Bay Area Patient Sample (at the time of the first interview, late 1957–early 1958)

Woman	Husband	Children	Marital Status	Napa
Shirley Arlen (26)	James (24)	M—5 months M—19 months	Married 2 years	36 weeks ECT[a]
Joan Baker (35)	Arnold (41)	F—12 F—7	Married 15 years; Arnold left	18 weeks ECT
Irene James (40)	Ralph (46)	F—7	Married 9 years; her second	15 weeks ECT
Wanda Karr (29)	Richard (28)	F—2 F—2 weeks	Married 3 years	8 weeks ECT
Eve Low (38)	Chester (38)	F—10 M—7 F—2	Married 13 years	11 weeks ECT
June Mark (33)	Paul (34)	F—11 F—8 F—4	Married 12 years; her second	12 weeks ECT
Joyce Noon (26)	Mel (37)	M—7	Married 2 years; living together 8 years; his third, her second	7 weeks
Louise Oren (30)	Jack (32)	M—11 F—3	Married 9 years; son/illegitimate adopted by Jack	9 weeks
Rose Price (34)	William (46)	M—13 M—11 M—4	Married 14 years	8 weeks

TABLE 1.1 *(continued)*

Woman	Husband	Children	Marital Status	Napa
Ruth Quinn (38)	Tim (36)	M—13 F—11	Married 14 years; Tim left	5 months ECT
Ann Rand (36)	Louis (37)	M—16 M—11 M—6	Son/previous marriage; married 13 years, her second	6 weeks
Peggy Sand (29)	Floyd (36)	F—11 F—6	Married 13 years	19 weeks
Cora Thorne (31)	Peter (31)	F—7 M—5 M—11 mo.	Married 9 years; Peter left/later reconciled	29 weeks ECT
Donna Urey (26)	Albert (27)	F—8 M—7 M—6 M—6 F—3	Married 8 years	64 weeks ECT
Rita Vick (29)	Leo (36)	M—2 M—1	Married 3 years; living together 6 years; his second, her third; Rita/6 other children	13 weeks ECT
Kate White (36)	Nelson (38)	F—5 F—2	Married 12 years	29 weeks
Mary Yale (29)	George (34)	F—4	Married 5 years	18 weeks ECT

[a]The abbreviation "ECT" indicates that electroconvulsive therapy was applied to the patient during hospitalization.

marriage (Berger and Kellner 1970) provide the foundation for order-ing everyday life. As Peter Berger and Hansfried Kellner comment, this life-ordering aspect of the family has its roots in the "broader configura-tions of our society," especially the "crystallization of a so-called private sphere of existence, more and more segregated from the immediate controls of the public institutions . . . and yet defined and utilized as the main social arena for the industrial revolution and its consequences" (1970, 55).

This structuring aspect of family life is independent of gender; but its components are essentially determined by gender. Another historically grounded "broader configuration of our society," and one that affects the response to trouble, is the distribution of the "internal" and "external" social "economy of the family" between the genders (Goffman 1971). Woman's place in the family, in the fifties, was one of responsibility for the internal economy, or household; man's place was external, in the workplace. Thus, these families' experience with the women's schizo-phrenia and hospitalization was profoundly shaped by gender.

Madness in the family threatens the members' sense of order, of stable selves, and of the other's proper place (Goffman 1971). For women in the fifties their "place" was restricted to the household and their roles as wife and mother. The threat of mental illness to woman's place, therefore, was a threat to the essential order of life: to the private order of the family, and (since, as Berger and Kellner note, the private sphere has come to be fundamentally ordering of the public) to the external social order (Chesler 1972; Schur 1984). Hospitalization unbalances the practical economy of the family, just as schizophrenia shakes its nomic founda-tions. When married men in the fifties were hospitalized, their wives were left without a provider (Yarrow et al. 1955). When married women were hospitalized, their families were left without a housewife. There was no one to wash the dishes, sweep the floor, or take the children to school.

Madness in the family also threatens love. Some of the Bay Area men and women said that they loved each other; others said that love had gone or had never been there. It is difficult to love someone and call them

TABLE 1.2

Bay Area Spouses' Marital Happiness Ratings (at the time of the original study) and Follow-up Outcomes

Name	Marital Happiness Rating[a]	Outcome in 1972
Shirley Arlen	Extremely unhappy; conflictful	Still married
Joan Baker	Extremely unhappy; conflictful	Divorced
Irene James	Reasonably happy	Still married
Wanda Karr	Reasonably happy	Still married
Eve Low	Rocky; one said good, the other not	Still married
June Mark	Reasonably happy	Divorced—Mrs. Mark later died
Joyce Noon	Extremely unhappy; conflictful	Still married
Louise Oren	Very good	Still married
Rose Price	Reasonably happy	Divorced
Ruth Quinn	Extremely unhappy; conflictful	Divorced
Ann Rand	Rocky; one said good, the other not	Still married—Mrs. Rand later died
Peggy Sand	Extremely unhappy; conflictful	Still married
Cora Thorne	Rocky; one said good, the other not	Still married
Donna Urey	Rocky; one said good, the other not	Still married
Rita Vick	Generally unsatisfactory	Divorced
Kate White	Rocky; one said good, the other not	Divorced
Mary Yale	Reasonably happy	Divorced

[a]Unless specified, both marital partners agreed on the same rating on a five-point scale: Very good, reasonably happy; rocky (one said good, the other not); generally unsatisfactory; extremely unhappy.

mad, although it is also difficult to love someone and overlook their distress. The original researchers, recognizing the significance of emotions in the processes they sought to understand, asked the Bay Area couples to rate their marital happiness, using a five-choice scale. Table 1.2 displays the results, and also indicates whether the couples were still married by the time of the 1972 follow-up interviews.

The processes of schizophrenia and hospitalization, then, were shaped by the nature of the fifties family: by its gender-role structure, by its essential privacy, by its nomic functions, and by the feelings that were shared between the members. But despite the primacy of the private, these families were part of a larger social structure and of a web of social institutions. Psychiatric hospitalization subjected the Bay Area women to the mental-health legislation prevailing in the fifties and to current treatments. And for married women patients, the effect of mental health legislation in the fifties was to reinforce the patriarchal authority of the husband with the medical authority of the (usually male) psychiatrist.

This study is cultural and interactional in emphasis, as well as structural and historical. The legal and diagnostic procedures by which the Bay Area women were committed to Napa had their origins in family interactions, through and by which the women came to be seen by themselves and others as troubled and in need of help. Robert Emerson and Sheldon Messinger (1977), in their analysis of trouble in interaction, point out that in our culture what comes eventually to be crystallized as schizophrenia begins with someone's sense that something is wrong, someone is troubled, and something needs to be done about it. Only through these interaction processes do wives become madwives and mental patients.

The classic interactionist study of mental illness and hospitalization is Erving Goffman's *Asylums*, which was written at about the time the Bay Area women were patients at Napa (1961). Both Napa and the New York setting for *Asylums* were state hospitals, and both were in some ways like small cities. Large enough to develop social institutions and inmate cultures, they were in some ways richer cultural milieus than traditional fifties families (the consequences of this irony for the women's experience in Napa will be discussed in chapter 4). Indeed, my analysis of the female mental patient's moral career focuses on the meaning of this experience in the context of the woman's place in the traditional family rather than in the bureaucratic context of staff–patient interaction. It is in this area that the intensive interview method can make its particular contribution, as opposed to the participant observation characteristic of standard mental-hospital ethnographies (Goffman 1961; Perruci 1974).

Family and Gender Roles in the Fifties

The families in the Bay Area study were in some ways, though not in others, representatives of the standard fifties family. They were typical in the value they placed on having and raising children, in their belief in marriage and the family as social institutions (even among those respondents contemplating divorce), and in their gender-role relationships. The man's job was to go to work and bring home the paycheck; the woman's was to guide its consumption, do housework and "emotion work" (Hochschild 1983), and bear and raise children.

The Bay Area families were formed by what Glenn Elder has called the "children of the Depression" of the 1920s and 1930s (1974). For reasons both social-psychological (Elder 1974) and demographic-economic (Easterlin 1968), this postwar cohort threw themselves into the business of marrying and having children as no twentieth-century generation has done before or since. The fifties had a birth rate higher than either the decade before or the two and a half decades after, a divorce rate lower than these two periods, and an earlier age at marriage than before or afterward (Cherlin 1981). Although the majority of married women were not, in the fifties, part of the labor force, the percentage of women with preschool children who worked outside the home rose from

11 percent to 19 percent between 1949 and 1959. Cherlin says of the fifties:

After nearly a decade of depression and four terrible years of war, Americans finally had prosperity as they entered the 1950s. And, except for the more limited Korean conflict, they finally had peace. Millions of men and women had been forced to postpone marrying during the hard times of the 1930s and the austerity and separation brought about by the war. . . . What was surprising was that years after this pent-up demand for marriage and children should have been satisfied, the birth and marriage rates remained high. As late as 1957 the Bureau of the Census estimated that nearly half of all young women who would ever marry would do so before they reached age 20. Moreover the annual birth rate rose steadily in the 1950s, reaching its peak in 1957. . . . Looking back now at the 1950s we can see how unusual this pattern of marriage and childrearing was. (1981, 34–35)

The meaning of family life in the fifties was different from that of earlier or later decades, within an economic and demographic context that favored getting married and having children (ibid.). The new fifties families began to populate the ever-expanding suburbs—such as those in the Bay Area of California—with their newfound ability to purchase single-family homes (ibid., 35). Even quite low-income people like the Bay Area respondents could buy and sell homes with relative ease. And once they were married and had children and homes, fifties Americans tended to place an extremely high value on these things (ibid., 36).

The imagery of the typical American family, which can still be found today, comes from the family of the fifties, despite its relative historical peculiarity. The traditional American family is nuclear and intact, and may not be part of extended community-kinship networks. It is patriarchal in the sense that male domination and female (and child) submission is assured by the division of labor in the family and in the society as a whole. Although it is structurally rare today, it remains a highly potent vision of the American ideal for many. And in the fifties, in the society as a whole and in the Bay Area families, it was a widespread reality.

SOCIOECONOMIC STATUS

The original researchers note that there was considerable variation in their respondents' socioeconomic status, but that "most cases fell into the upper-lower or lower middle classes" (Sampson et al. 1964, 14). They add that most of the families had incomes of less than $7,000 a year, but one had more than $15,000. All but one wife had at least some high-school education, and five had gone to college for a time or had teacher training. Three of the husbands had only grammar-school education; four had gone to college, and two of these had received degrees beyond the B.A. (ibid.).

The respondent families ranged from what might be considered the unrespectable poor to the middle class. In the first category were the Prices, who lived in a dirty, rat-infested home belonging to the company for which Mr. Price worked in an unskilled, blue-collar job. Neither Price had finished high school. In the latter category were the Whites, who both had some college education (he had an M.A.) and who had both, in earlier periods of their lives, engaged in professional-level work. Two or three of the families could be classified as working-class poor, while a few were middle class; the remainder of the sample, as the original researchers judged, fell between these extremes.

In other ways, however, the lives of most respondents exhibited considerable structural similarities that are characteristic of the lower- to lower-middle-class household in fifties American society. They were all traditional households. Although some had close contact with one or two relatives who lived in the home or nearby, few were integrated into stable kin networks, perhaps because they had originally come from places other than the Bay Area. Most of the couples, in fact, had lived in the area for less than five years.

In the years preceding the study, the families had had a history of marital instability; five of the wives and two of the husbands had previously been married, several more than once. A number of the Bay Area marriages had been contracted on the spur of the moment, after only a few hours' or days' acquaintance. There was also a history of instability in

these respondents' families of origin, with at least half of the sample
reporting close relatives who had spent time in mental hospitals (as had
two of the sample husbands). Three of the wives had in the past lost
custody of one or more of their children.

The lives of the Bay Area respondents were characterized by considerable stress. None of the families felt that they had adequate money to
live on, and all of them worried (some continually) about paying their
bills. While a number of the husbands had steady, full-time employment, for about half the families the husbands' employment was sporadic, punctuated by worrisome periods of unemployment—and this at
a time of relative ease in obtaining many levels of job in the U.S.
economy and in the Bay Area. Both the husbands and the wives in this
study cited the financial stress of bills or unemployment as one of the
factors that precipitated the wives' hospitalization.

One aspect of their lives that was less of a problem than it would be
today was housing; although their finances were often unstable, these
families could and did find housing that they could afford in a rental
market that was much more open in the fifties than it is in the eighties.
Indeed, more than half of these financially troubled respondents owned
or bought their own homes during the period of the research, while the
majority moved, some of them several times, during the study, seeking
better living conditions in the open market. Those respondents who did
own their own homes focused on them as a source of leisure activity and
personal gratification. While the women ran the household on an everyday basis, the husbands spent the weekend either "puttering around" or
engaged in major renovation projects in the home, sometimes persuad-
ing the other family members (and even, on occasion, the handy researcher) to join in.

These families' life-styles also seemed uninteresting—at least to some
of the original interviewers, and sometimes, in reflective moments, to
themselves. Most, though not all, families were isolated from frequent
social contacts either from relatives or from friends and centered their
lives around the family home. Within this context of familial isolation,
the women were individually isolated during their husbands' working

hours, a factor that many of them understood as precipitating their emotional difficulties (see chapter 3). Few of the families either could afford to, or seemed motivated to, engage in social activities outside the home, with occasional exceptions related either to churchgoing or to camping expeditions. Life revolved, as it does for many families today, around the TV set.

Mental Illness and the Law in the Fifties

While the treatment of deviance has been largely in the hands of medical professionals throughout the twentieth century, psychiatric diagnoses, treatment, and mental-health laws were somewhat different in the fifties than they are in the eighties. The diagnosis of schizophrenia was applied in the fifties to a greater range of behaviors than is seen as appropriate in the eighties. Electroconvulsive therapy, the treatment of choice for schizophrenics in the state hospitals of the fifties, is no longer seen as suitable for them. And the laws governing involuntary commitment to and release from state hospitals have moved in the direction of greater attentiveness to the rights of would-be mental patients.

According to contemporary anthropological and historical scholarship, the notion of craziness or madness has existed through all recorded cultures, as a conceptual category used to describe bizarre, inexplicable behavior (Murphy 1976; Horwitz 1982b). The specific behavior defined as mad, of course, varies according to time and place. The notion of mental illness, or the medical model of madness, has a history as long as Western civilizaton. Peter Conrad and Joseph Schneider describe the coexistence of medical and lay interpretations of madness:

The Greeks had two explanations for madness. The cosmological-supernatural explanation—that madness was a possession caused by the gods or inflicted by the spirit underworld—was believed by most of the Greek populace. It made sense, since the mythological gods were considered part of everyday life. The natural-medical explanation, the first elaborated medical explanation in recorded history, which defined madness as a disease with natural causes seems to have been adopted only by certain segments of the upper classes. Greek medicine . . . [saw] madness as a disease with the same etiology as somatic diseases. (1980, 39–40)

Thomas Scheff argues that contemporary explanations for madness take the form of common-sense stereotypes, learned in childhood, which are overlaid by—but not replaced by—medical conceptions learned in adulthood (1966, 64–67). However, his discussion highlights the fact that for us, unlike the ancient Greeks, everyday life and medical concepts have merged; spirits, gods, and mythologies, as explanations for madness, are no longer viable.

The Bay Area respondents indicated their sense of this historical progression by referring to a contemporary "greater understanding" of mental illness on the part of the general population. In fact, studies of the general population itself indicate that people are willing to interpret even more behavior as indicative of mental illness than they were in the fifties (Conrad and Schneider 1980, 59). The pervasiveness of the mental-illness model of madness, its stratification by social class and education, and some of its functions in everyday life are indicated by Nelson White, husband of one of the Bay Area women:

He felt that his wife was somewhat concerned about the stigma of having been in a booby hatch. It was true that the neighbors were more enlightened about mental illness, most of them were professionals and had a good deal of education. He commented that education did not necessarily mean they were more intelligent, but they probably understood the fact that mental illness was an illness you can get just like any other one.

The entrenchment of the medical model of madness during the past century and a half has been accompanied by a progressive specialization of practice and specificity of diagnosis, as has also been the case in general medicine. The set of behaviors identified in the fifties (and today in modified form) as schizophrenia was first subject to classification and naming in the nineteenth century (Barham 1984). Diagnostic processes in both general and psychiatric medicine are historically grounded. As indicated in the third edition of the *Diagnostic and Statistical Manual of Mental Disorders* (American Psychiatric Association 1980):

The first [1952] edition of the American Psychiatric Association's *Diagnostic and Statistical Manual of Mental Disorders* . . . was the first official manual of mental disorders to contain a glossary of descriptions of the diagnostic categories. The use of the term "reaction" throughout the classification reflected the influence of Adolf Meyer's psychological view that mental disorders represented reactions of the personality to psychological, social, and biological factors. (1980, 1)

The first edition says of "Schizophrenic Reactions": "The term is synonymous with the formerly used term dementia praecox. It represents a group of psychotic reactions characterized by fundamental disturbances in reality relationships and concept formations, with affective, behavioral and intellectual disturbances in various degrees and mixtures" (1952, 26).

The various etiological theories of schizophrenia that exist today originated in the late nineteenth and early twentieth centuries and have waxed and waned in popularity since: the somatic biochemical, genetic, and other physiological theories, and the psychological theories based on family pathology (Holzman 1977).

During the fifties both biochemical and family-based theories of schizophrenia were current in the state hospitals, with a particular interest in the "schizophrenogenic family" or "schizophrenogenic mother" (Johnston and Planansky 1968). At Napa, the emergency admitting diagnosis was made by whatever psychiatrist was in attendance; the patient was subsequently evaluated by teams of doctors, nurses, and social workers. What is most interesting about these formal admission and discharge conferences, as will be seen in subsequent chapters, is the degree to which the diagnostic process was influenced by gender and by the woman's place in the traditional family.

TREATMENT

The treatments applied to the Bay Area patients at Napa were typical of those in the fifties state hospitals: electroconvulsive therapy (ECT, EST, or Shock, which ten of the seventeen patients received), drug therapy, hydrotherapy, and the various therapies that involve doing or talking, such as occupational therapy (OT) and group therapy. Insulin injections or other means to induce seizures besides electricity were used in hospitals in the fifties, but not at Napa.

ECT was the most significant treatment in the context of gender and family relationships (to be discussed in greater detail in chapter 5). It involves inducing epileptic seizures through the application of electrical current to the brain, either unilaterally (at the center of the forehead) or bilaterally (on both temples). Although the use of electricity in medicine has a long history, with folk origins in Western culture, its modern application began in the 1930s with the claim of a Hungarian asylum superintendent that schizophrenia could not coexist with epilepsy in an organism; inducing epileptic seizures in schizophrenics, he reasoned, would cure the disorder (Alexander and Selesnick 1966). From the thirties to the mid-sixties, ECT was commonly used in the state hospitals for the treatment of schizophrenia.

A second, physiologically based therapy used in psychiatric medicine for at least three centuries is hydotherapy: the use of cold sedative tubs or wet packs of sheets to control and calm patients. In their participant observation study of a private mental hospital in the early fifties, A. Stanton and M. Schwartz described the use of "cold packs" as "a hydro-therapeutic measure: patients are wrapped closely in cold wet sheets; after a few minutes, the patient becomes flushed and warm, he is quieted and often goes to sleep" (1954, 127). They noted, as have many observers since, that hydrotherapy is among the repertoire of medical-model "cures" that can readily be adapted to organizational control requirements: "seclusion, cold wet sheet packs and sedative medication . . . were prescribed officially as 'treatment' which was to be given to a patient only when expected to be beneficial to him. But at the same time they were used also as measures of social restraint" (ibid.).

Treatment of patients by the use of major tranquilizers or psychoactive drugs became more and more commonplace in the state hospitals during the sixties and seventies, gradually replacing ECT as the treatment of choice. All but two of the Bay Area women reported to the interviewers that they had been given some sort of drug treatment while at Napa. Although many of the women could not name the drugs they were given, at least at first, those who could cited sparine, vesperin, and occasionally thorazine.

Finally, the state hospitals of the fifties used therapies grounded in routine activities on the ward, such as the "reality therapy" of ward housework, and the making of potholders in OT. In addition, patients were engaged in group therapy of a sort that mixed issues of patient psychopathology with those of patient misbehavior on the ward. None of the women received individual psychotherapy prior to discharge from Napa.

MENTAL-HEALTH LAW

Of the seventeen women in this study, six were first admitted to Napa as voluntary patients and eleven as involuntary. Of the six volunteers, one (Peggy Sand) was committed involuntarily by her husband to the county hospital immediately after her release from the state hospital. In the California of 1957 to 1961, persons could sign their spouses into the psychiatric hospital if they also obtained the signature of one licensed physician (who need not be, as is the case today, a psychiatrist). In the judicial review of the commitment process, it was the spouse's wishes and views on the matter of the patient's mental illness that were consulted. In addition, the patient after release could be recommitted at the spouse's

behest. These procedures inverted the prevailing order of familial control for wives' commitment of mentally disordered men, but magnified
it in the case of committed women.

During the period of the original study there were nine state hospitals
in California (plus Atascadero, a facility for the criminally insane). Napa
was one of six in northern California. The popular view of the state
hospitals of the fifties and sixties as populated by very long-term patients
was not true for first admissions, either for the Bay Area women or for the
California hospital population in general. About two-thirds of first
admissions to California state mental hospitals in the late fifties were
released after more than six months but less than one year (Bardach
1972, 41). By the end of the Bay Area follow-up period (a total of thirty-
six months), none of the sample remained at Napa on their first admission (though five had been readmitted between one and six times).

The Bay Area women were typical of state hospital patients of the
fifties in that they were married women. In a survey of all schizophrenic
first admissions to California state hospitals in 1953 and 1954, the
researchers found that 55 percent of women patients were married at the
time of admission, compared with 29 percent of men. Twenty-four
percent of the women patients and 18 percent of the male patients were
divorced, separated, or widowed (Sampson et al. 1964, 21). The majority of first admissions to state hospitals in the fifties were women. In that
decade in California, release from the state mental hospital was a graduated process, which began with visits from the family and then progressed to visits to the family for periods of time ranging from twenty-
four hours to ten days. Following a discharge conference, the outcome
might be a return to hospitalization, a leave of absence, or (more rarely)
an unconditional discharge. If a leave of absence was granted, the ex-
patient remained in a sort of "probationary" status for one year, in
which she could be returned to hospital by her spouse (or other guardian) at any time.

Even with such a small sample there was considerable variation
among the Bay Area patients with respect to symptom severity. At least
eleven of the women exhibited the delusions, hallucinations, and bizarre

behaviors typical of those whom the lay person would classify as "crazy" and the psychiatrist as "schizophrenic." At the other end of the spectrum, Peggy Sand appeared to be suffering from little more than marital and role stress on admission to Napa. The remainder fell somewhere between these two extremes. A 1972 reanalysis of the Bay Area case histories indicated a greater hesitation, fifteen years later, for psychiatrists to use the "schizophrenic" label (these diagnoses were made by a team of sociologists and psychologists from the University of California, Berkeley):

Shirley Arlen: "Definitely not" schizophrenic; "no symptoms." Probably reactive depression or adult adjustment problems. Not psychotic. On rehospitalization after the first episode Mrs. Arlen was diagnosed as "neurotic depression."

Joan Baker: "Probably not" schizophrenic. There is only flimsy evidence of hallucinations. "Probably not psychotic. Obviously depressed, maybe hysterical personality."

Irene James: "Uncertain." The initial problem is vague—there is weak evidence of paranoia, she was very preoccupied with her delusions. On rehospitalization she was diagnosed "involutional."

Wanda Karr: "Uncertain. The primary symptoms are withdrawal, anger, and perhaps some delusions. Psychotic episode."

Eve Low: "Probably" schizophrenic; a psychotic episode, paranoid, delusional, and expressed ideas of reference; quite incoherent.

June Mark: "Probably schizophrenic. The initial onset is less clearly schizophrenic than the outcome. She was obviously absorbed with her children and paranoid."

Joyce Noon: "Definitely" schizophrenic. "Hallucinations cap a lifetime of pathology."

Louise Oren: "Uncertain" diagnosis; primary feature seems to be anxious delusions. Psychotic episode? On rehospitalization diagnosed "acute psychoneurosis."

Rose Price: "Uncertain. She appears to be another of the inadequate persons characterized by withdrawal and grossly impaired functioning. Possibly psychotic."

Ruth Quinn: "Probably" schizophrenic. Paranoid and delusional.

Ann Rand: "Uncertain. Generally she appears anxious and depressed. Just prior to admission she was delusional in a bizarre manner. Psychotic episode." On rehospitalization diagnosed manic depressive.

Peggy Sand: "Definitely not" schizophrenic. "Possibly a hysterical personality but no psychosis."

Cora Thorne: "Probably not" schizophrenic. "Paranoia and delusions very likely linked to depression." On rehospitalization diagnosed involutional.

Donna Urey: "Definitely" schizophrenic. "Long periods of hallucination, wandering away from home topped off by arson."

Rita Vick: "Probably not" schizophrenic. "There is a lifelong pattern of insane rages but no evidence of functional or affective psychosis. Only hint of thought disorder is confusion and some bizarreness—selling furniture. Character disorder."

Kate White: "Uncertain. She had some delusions, was preoccupied with guilt and concern for her children. Psychotic episode."

Mary Yale: "Definitely not" schizophrenic. "She probably was not psychotic. . . . The only symptoms appear to be excessive dependency, protectiveness, and some preoccupation with her sexual identity. Personality disorder."

If these diagnoses were reconsidered in the late 1980s they would once again be altered. As appendix A indicates, at least three of the women—Mrs. Rand, Mrs. Quinn, and Mrs. Baker—had problems with over- or underweight that today would classify them as suffering from "eating disorders."

The Moral Career
of the Mental Patient

Within the historical context of the fifties and early sixties (but not attending directly to this context), Erving Goffman developed his theory of the "moral career" of the mental patient. He uses the term to stress what he sees as the "moral aspects of career—that is, the regular sequence of changes that career entails in the person's self and in his framework of imagery for judging himself and others" (1961, 130). He sees the patient's moral career as a sequence of phases: "the [prepatient] period prior to entering the hospital . . . the inpatient phase; [and] the period of discharge from the hospital, should this occur, namely, the expatient phase" (ibid., 130–131).

The moral career of the mental patient is embedded not only in the bureaucratic context of a hospital but also in a society, a culture, and a network of social institutions. The relationship between a particular society and the moral career of the mental patient is a reflexive one, with the career both embedded in and influenced by the typical courses of everyday life in that society. Thus, in the Bay Area study, the women's careers as mental patients influenced, and were influenced by, their careers as housewives and mothers in the traditional fifties family.

THE PREPATIENT PHASE:
Trouble and Its Interpretation

The prepatient phase of the moral career begins with an amorphous set of troubles and ends with the process of commitment to a mental hospital. Analyzing the process of defining, redefining, and taking action concerning the respondents' individual and marital troubles, Emerson and Messinger developed a theory of trouble that they refer to as the "micro-politics" of trouble in interaction (1977). These micropolitics precipitate the prepatient into the patient phase of the moral career.

To some extent the micropolitics of trouble in our society is shaped by assumptions common to the culture and independent of gender; for example, that trouble is something that should be attended to, and that personal troubles and troubles in interpersonal relations can have medical interpretations. However, it is clear from the data on schizophrenic individuals and their spouses (see also Yarrow et al. 1955; Warren 1983) that interpretation of troubles is heavily dependent on historically structured gender and marital roles. This intersection of trouble and gender is the focus of my analysis.

Emerson and Messinger see the trouble process as having a natural history, one that begins with "a vague sense of something wrong on the part of someone in a given interaction or relationship" (1977, 121). They explore the questions of definition and remedial action involved in the trouble theories that begin with this vague notion, both when "parties outside the trouble are mobilized around it" and "when those outsiders' involvement rests on formal authority rather than personalities" (ibid.). The moral career of the mental patient crystallizes when specifically medical, then psychiatric, authorities are brought into what was previously private marital trouble. Once trouble has become defined as more than accidental or situational—once it can no longer be explained away—"a remedy is sought and applied, it works temporarily or not at all, then some new remedy is sought" (ibid., 122). Consequently—or at times simultaneously—"trouble is progressively elaborated, analyzed, and specified as to type and cause" (ibid.).

This study focuses on what Emerson and Messinger call "relational troubles—that is, those in which remedial efforts are addressed to another in a recognized relationship with the troubled person. . . . unlike efforts to remedy personal troubles, trying to resolve relational troubles raises issues concerning the distribution of rights and responsibilities in that relationship" (ibid., 123). Typically, the first line of remedy in relational troubles is the intrinsic remedy, in which one party tries directly to change the behavior of the other. Such initial complaints are met with varying degrees of success, and are often only the beginning of "an extended remedial cycle," in which a variety of behavior-changing strategies are attempted. During this cycle, past actions may be retrospectively interpreted as leading up to the trouble. Eventually, an organized and organizing theory of the stages of the trouble and attempts at remedy may be formulated by the offended party (ibid., 124–125). One solution for the aggrieved or offended party in a marriage is to terminate the relationship. But where this strategy is not used, for whatever reason, "troubles and remedial strategies greatly increase in complexity. Under such circumstances, pressures to seek outside remedies often accelerate" (ibid., 126). Outside parties are brought or allowed into the process of trouble definition and handling once intrinsic remedies have been judged a failure: "Critical involvement emerges when the third party directly intervenes and establishes a relationship with the troubled parties, who thus no longer deal exclusively with one another. With this event the remedies considered are no longer intrinsic, but extrinsic to the troubled relationship" (ibid.).

Initial troubleshooters or remedial agents are generally close friends or relatives of at least one of those involved in the troubled relationship. From these third parties, the search for definitions and remedies may expand to include official social-control or therapeutic agents—ministers, marriage counselors, police, or psychiatrists. If the troubles are perceived as medical rather than, say, criminal or spiritual, the remedial agent chosen may be a psychiatrist or psychologist. Close friends may define the problem as medical and convince the troubled parties to approach the medical establishment with their problems (ibid., 127–128).

Once external remedies are sought within officialdom, the issue of power enters the situation. In a previous section, I discussed the asymmetrical role structure of the fifties family, with the husband's control balanced by the wife's dependence. Family troubleshooters can try to influence the remedial process, but they do not have final authority in the matter. Psychiatrists and psychologists, however, especially when teamed with police and the court system, do have such authority. Once the remedial process includes officials, women become subject to the dual control of husbands and of experts, while the remedial authority of experts over people in general draws, in the case of women (and children), on familial authority as well.

From the perspective of the prepatient, the injection of psychiatric expertise into his or her life represents a form of betrayal by intimate family members. The patient experiences an "alienative coalition" of family members and experts, who construct a betrayal funnel of conspiratorial events through which she passes from her home to the mental hospital. Although natural histories have a common structure, Emerson and Messinger point out that the definition of trouble and the remedies attempted vary in at least two ways. They depend on prior histories of trouble and their resolution within the relationship; and they depend on the social context of the relationship:

Such factors as the kinds of controls and remedies available in the particular social situation, the availability of limitations upon their use, the presence and strength of ties with outside parties and possible troubleshooters, and the degree of legitimacy accorded each outsider's potential involvement in the troubled situation, all shape not only the nature of initial efforts to respond to the trouble within the relationship, but also the occasion and nature of outside intervention. (ibid., 126–127)

One of the features of trouble interpretation to be elaborated here is the gender dynamics of the marital relationship, set within the historical context of the structure of marriage in the fifties.

THE PATIENT PHASE:
Psychiatric Transformation

Goffman's analysis of the patient phase of the moral career (1961) focuses on the development of the patient role in interaction with the mental hospital's staff and on the various transformations of self that attend this process. He notes the ceremony of "identity stripping" by which the new mental patient is shorn of her or his former identity both symbolically and materially (the Bay Area women had to surrender their wedding rings upon admission), and the labeling process by which the self is reconstituted into the sick role.

My analysis differs from Goffman's in that the focus is on the meaning of mental hospitalization in the context of the patient's overall life, rather than on the interactions by which roles and selves are transformed. This difference is related in part to differences in method: the ethnographic or observational method highlights meaningful interaction in situ, while intensive interviews bring into focus the meaning of the particular experience in a larger biographical context. The implication of this methodological difference is that not only are staff–patient interactions significant in understanding the impact of hospitalization on social role, but also the patient's preexisting social relationships—not only the transformed self, but also the historical self (Musgrove 1977).

The "historical self" refers to the self embedded in biography rather than the self transformed by the immediate social situation. In his intensive-interview studies of religious converts, chronic patients, and others, Frank Musgrove found that they saw themselves not only as religious, sick, or other selves expressive of their immediate environment, but also as historical selves. Within the framework of the historical self, the institutional role was only one expression or permutation of an entire life course (ibid.). I examine the patient phase of the moral career as it reflects the biographical context of the sick role.

This is not to say that the Bay Area women, or patients in general, did not or do not undergo changes while they are hospitalized. But changes in the self and in social relationships while at Napa were a consequence not only of hospitalization and of staff–patient interaction, but also of the interaction of the patient with nonstaff others. In the original study, the patients' significant others included mothers, mothers-in-law, friends, siblings, offspring—"over one hundred direct informants, not counting state hospital personnel." (Sampson et al. 1964, 13)—and, most importantly, husbands. Analysis of the changing self of the hospitalized madwife begins with the nature of her relationship with her husband, just as her everyday life is encompassed within the family. Only in this context can the meaning of patienthood to the madwife be understood.

THE EX-PATIENT PHASE:
Restoration and Stigma

Although Sampson, Messinger, and Towne (1964) do not analyze the patient phase of the moral career, they attend to the ex-patient and prepatient phases. Their concern in *Schizophrenic Women* is with the adjustment these women and their families made on returning to the same familial situation that had precipitated the original crisis. My analysis of the ex-patient phase of the moral career is framed by the traditional gender-role relationship within the family, in which the woman attains much of her sense of self from performance of household and child-care duties. My interest is, specifically, in the way an ex-patient's sense of role competence or incompetence depends on the structure of the fifties family as well as in the former patient's experiences when returned to the family. More generally, I seek to discover how a sense of proper self is recovered from the feeling of stigma attached to the hospital experience.

In Goffman's classic analysis (1963), stigmatization refers to negative reactions to those who possess culturally devalued attributes. Being an ex-mental patient is what Goffman refers to as a "discrediting" stigma, one that is not immediately apparent—as is, say, physical handicap—

but which, if discovered, can lead to negative stereotyping and distressing encounters. Further, stigmatization can affect the ex-patient's opportunities, as it did in the case of some of the Bay Area women: during the initial year after release, the women were still legally classified as incompetent and were not permitted to drive a car, vote in elections, or sign contracts without the permission of spouses and state officials. Thus, the definition and handling of trouble takes on a different cast in the ex-patient as against the prepatient phase of family and community life. Once labeled, a person's subsequent history takes on a predictable course. Messinger notes:

the patient role defines your qualities in a more or less permanent way that is independent of continuing contact with the patient role . . . to some extent independent of your current and future performances, too, and that's the rub. Once in you are for evermore potentially psychotic in a way untrue of others. The way next of relations, mediators, etc. have been trained to interpret the trouble you create in this wise. Your record is with you. (n.d., 21)

The fifties ex-patient was monitored by her closest relative or spouse for signs of trouble recurrence and was liable to have her actions interpreted as symptoms of mental illness. Furthermore, the coalition between spouse and social worker or psychiatrist continued in this phase, since the overseer was instructed to bring the individual back in at the "first signs" of trouble. Ideally, as Messinger notes, the ex-patient would have internalized the sick role enough to readmit herself with little prompting: "just as the attempt is to seduce the prepatient into making the steps (to mental hospitalization) without trouble on the way in, so the attempt is to seduce her to make the reentrance steps smooth. Ideally she will initiate action" (ibid., 2). It is part of the future fate of the ex-patient that her troubles can no longer be encompassed within a general theory of trouble, but are now perceived in psychiatric terms.

History and Social Change

I have shown how the individual experiences of these madwives and their families are embedded in the historical context of the fifties and in the social context of the patients' moral careers, and have indicated the ways in which theoretical and methodological transformations in disciplinary understandings affect contemporary interpretations of historical data. But it is also important to take note of those areas of experience that have some parallel in the contemporary situation of institutionalized housewives. To that end I will indicate some of the changes that have occurred in the structure of the family, mental-health law, and psychiatry since the late fifties and their relevance to the hospitalized housewife.

THE FAMILY AND GENDER ROLES
SINCE THE FIFTIES

A number of the family's structural features described earlier began to change in the sixties. The overall decline in the birthrate that has characterized most of the twentieth century resumed. The steep rise in the divorce rate with which we are all familiar began in 1962; nine of every thousand married women over the age of fifteen were divorced in 1960, as compared with twenty-two of every thousand in 1980 (Cherlin 1974, 22). By 1980, 60 percent of married women with children were in the labor force.

Although the structure of the family has changed profoundly since the early sixties, much of the meaning and imagery associated with it has not. Indeed, many scholars argue that there has been no real structural change, on the grounds that our society remains—as it was in the fifties—capitalist in social form, with a relatively intact gender division of labor. With Rae André (1981), Heidi Hartmann suggests that the control men exert over women in the marital relationship and the dependence engendered in women are related to "the differences in material interests among family members that are caused by their differing relations to patriarchy and capitalism" (1981, 369). She asserts that this control–dependency situation is experienced in everyday marital interaction through housework, by which men seek relief from household and child-rearing tasks by passing them on to women (ibid., 372).

The functionalist view is that the division of labor between women and men into household maintenance and extrahousehold production leads to a Durkheimian consensus in the family. By contrast, Hartmann argues that "the underlying concept of the family as an active agent with unified interests is erroneous, and I offer an alternative concept of the family as a locus of struggle" (ibid., 368). She locates the source of potential family trouble in the position of women itself—trouble that may find expression in marital conflicts over "the adequacy of paychecks versus the adequacy of housework" (ibid., 369).

I would argue that the family today is both nomic and ordering in the ways described above (Berger and Kellner 1970), and conflictual and alienating in the ways—and for the reasons—analyzed by Hartmann (1981). Marriage, in the twentieth-century capitalist state, provides the main ground for meaning and order, feeling and communication, the community of self and other. But at the same time marriage is unequal—and in the fifties it was even more so than it is today (Pleck 1985). The economic dependence of the wife in traditional relationships causes alienation as surely as does the economic dependence of workers who do not own the means of production. And this alienation separates the woman from the man and the woman from her own sense of herself.

Although there have been some changes in the economic place of women since the fifties, there has been less change in spheres of household labor, both physical and emotional. Despite the fact that participation in the work force by married women with young children has increased considerably since the fifties, the eighties woman's responsibility for household labor has not altered very much. In general, "husbands of wives who work for wages do not spend more time on housework than husbands whose wives do not work for wages" (Hartmann 1981, 379), although there is some evidence that between 1965 and 1975 time spent on housework fell between six hours a week for the "full time homemaker" and four hours a week for those with outside employment (ibid.). Statistics from 1976 indicate that full-time homemakers spent almost seventy hours a week in household work, including thirty in child care (ibid., 381). Pleck (1985) indicates that while "role overload" for working housewives (doing both an outside job and most housework) has declined since the seventies, women still do more of life's necessary labors than men.

The household role of married women has changed enough that the unique pressures of the fifties on women are clearly visible in the Bay Area interviews, but not enough that the experiences shared by these women have no parallels twenty or thirty years later. Walter Gove and Jeanette Tudor's description in 1973 of women's role (which they see as an explanation of higher rates of mental hospitalization among married women) would not read very differently had it been written decades earlier:

There are several reasons to assume that, because of the roles they typically occupy, women are more likely than men to have emotional problems. First, most women are restricted to a single major societal role—housewife—whereas most men occupy two such roles, household head and worker. . . . Second, it seems reasonable to assume that a large number of women find their major instrumental activities—raising children and keeping house—frustrating. (1973, 814)

The authors add that additional strain on women can come from the unstructured role of the housewife, which fosters both "brooding" and "letting things slide"; the low status of those jobs women do hold; and their generally diffuse expectations of the female role itself (see also Lopata 1971; Oakley 1974).

Phyllis Chesler summarizes several studies that investigate the relation between madness and the housewife, pointing out that schizophrenia is frequently discussed in terms of "sex role alienation or sex role rejection" and that female ex-patients tended to perform less well domestically than those never hospitalized. However, she also notes that the post-hospital "symptoms" experienced by ex-patients—feeling restless, worn out, tense, nervous, and grouchy—are also experienced by 47 to 60 percent of "normal" housewives (1972, 69).

The traditional housewife role contains the structural potential for going crazy, for feeling locked up, smothered, and unable to get out by any means short of madness (ibid.). Chesler describes the madness exit as it was experienced by a number of well-known women: "Fitzgerald, West and Plath were desperately and defiantly at odds with the female role. They attempted to escape its half-life by 'going crazy.' There, as helpless and self-destructive children, they were superficially freed from their female roles as private social losers, as wives and mothers." She adds that "Madness and asylums generally function as mirror images of the female experience and as penalties for being female as well as for desiring or daring not to be" (ibid., 39; see also Matthews 1984).

In addition to the performance of practical chores, housewifery involves what Arlie Russell Hochschild calls "emotion work" (1983). As Talcott Parsons (1951) indicated several decades ago, the gender divisions in the traditional family involve the woman in responsibility for the emotional, as well as the household, labor needed for the maintenance of family relationships. For the man, the family may be a "'relief zone' away from the pressures of work," but for the woman "it quietly imposes emotional obligations of its own" (Hochschild 1983, 32). According to Hochschild, the emotional work required of women is greater than that required of men, in the fifties as in the eighties.

As Hochschild also notes, one of the strongest types of emotional obligation is that of parent for child, especially that of mother for child (ibid., 69). A mother is not only supposed to take primary responsibility for the material care of her child, she is also supposed to take primary responsibility for emotional care (Margolis 1984). In the traditional family division of labor described—I think aptly for the eighties and fifties alike—by Talcott Parsons, the wife also has the primary, sometimes exclusive responsibility for family emotional work. Donna Urey described the troubles that led up to her hospitalization as originating in both her housewife and her mother roles (see chapters 2 and 3) and in the emotional work of her marriage: "at times he cared, and at other times he wouldn't, and I'd be the same way—I'd go along with his emotions. More or less, my emotions were set with his emotions; instead of having my own personal feelings I'd have his." In the type of marital bargain described in chapter 2, women like Mrs. Urey have traditionally understood their marital obligation in part as "emotion management [in] trade for economic support" (ibid., 20).

One aspect of emotional management is emotional labor, as Hochschild refers to it. Emotional labor requires one to "induce or suppress feeling in order to sustain the outward countenance that produces the proper state of mind in others" (ibid., 7). This description befits the Bay Area wives' accounts of the troubles that precipitated hospitalization, troubles that revolved around their sense of isolation and loneliness in the housewife role, the difficulties of housework and child care, and the lack of communication and intimacy in the marital relationship. Hochschild describes how workers can become "estranged or alienated from an aspect of self—either the body or the margins of the soul—that is used to do the work" (ibid.). For the housewife, both body and soul are involved in doing the household and emotional labor that cements the family—the traditional family of the fifties and the family in the newer world of the seventies and eighties, especially among the working class (Blumstein and Schwartz 1983).

One difference that would be expected among similarly situated women of the seventies and eighties would be at least a dim awareness that an anxiety response to the role of housewife could be a legitimate expression of structural strain rather than an idiosyncratic failure on the part of the emotionally unstable. But this difference may remain one only of potential. Helena Lopata says of the housewife that "society itself observes some of her difficulties, but usually evaluates them as a consequence of her 'neurotic' tendencies, 'underfeminine' attitudes, or 'selfish' traits. Sometimes she questions her personality, blaming herself rather than understanding the factors contributing to vague and inarticulate discontents" (1971, 34).

Nevertheless, feminist language is part of the cultural heritage of the eighties, and women situated similarly to the Bay Area subjects have access to that language. What was only a latent and ill-articulated sense of protest among the women of the fifties (Cherlin 1981; Matthews 1984) is today overt and well articulated, assisting individual women to formulate critiques of marital domination, unequal household and child-care roles, and female dependence. Madwives today have at least potentially a voice with which to protest the dismissal of their hopes, dreams, and burdens as instances of marital trouble and of mental-illness symptoms.

Mental Illness and the Law Since the Fifties

As indicated above, diagnostic processes have become more clearly specified and programmatic. The third edition of the *Diagnostic and Statistical Manual of Mental Disorders* comments that "Since in DSM-I [and] DSM-II . . . explicit criteria [for diagnosis] are not provided, the clinician is largely on his or her own in defining the content and boundaries of the diagnostic categories" (American Psychiatric Association 1980, 8). For making a diagnosis of schizophrenia (in one of its many subtypes), the *Manual* provides specific criteria for the duration and type of symptoms. In addition to "Deterioration from a previous level of functioning in such areas as work, social relations, and self-care" (ibid., 189), a schizophrenic diagnosis requires

At least one of the following . . . (1) bizarre delusions (content is patently absurd and has *no* possible basis in fact) . . . (2) somatic, grandiose, religious, nihilistic or other delusions . . . (3) delusions with persecutory or jealous content if accompanied by hallucinations of any type; (4) [and (5)] auditory hallucinations. . . . (6) incoherence, marked loosening of associations, markedly illogical thinking, or marked poverty of content of speech. (ibid., 188)

In response both to the expanded use of major tranquilizing drugs and to legislative intervention, the use of ECT in public psychiatric facilities declined considerably during the sixties and seventies. Recent data from California, however, indicate that the treatment is undergoing a resurgence there, this time in the private rather than the public mental-health sector (Warren 1987b).

Hydrotherapy is no longer used as a calming device in psychiatric hospitals. The major treatments in both public and private facilities today are drugs: phenothiazine in cases of schizophrenia and psychosis and others such as lithium carbonate for manic depression. The state hospitals continue to use the doing and talking therapies such as OT and group, and in addition many of them have set up family-therapy programs to deal with the involvement of the family system in the patient's emotional troubles.

Both mental-health law and the conditions and length of hospitalization have changed considerably in California (and in other states) since the fifties (Bardach 1972; Scull 1977; Warren 1982). California's current mental-health legislation, the Lanterman–Petris–Short Act (henceforth LPS) enacted in 1969, retains involuntary as well as voluntary confinement but requires considerably more due process than was necessary twenty or thirty years ago. Due process protections that exist today but did not in the fifties include prior written notification of all psychiatric–legal proceedings, the right to defense counsel in all judicial hearings, and the right to judicial review of psychiatric decisions through the writ of habeas corpus. Furthermore, discharge from involuntary commitment is absolute rather than conditional, with no provisions for a spouse to sign the ex-patient back in.

Under LPS (and similar legislation in other states), involuntary confinement is limited to fourteen days following an initial seventy-two hours for evaluation and treatment. After the fourteen-day period the commitment may be extended for varying lengths of time; in practice, the majority of patients are released after seventy-two hours plus fourteen days (Warren 1982). While the majority of state-hospital patients—both voluntary and involuntary—in the fifties were female, the majority in the eighties are male, although there are still more females in private hospitals than males. This change has come about in part because of the decline in the general state-hospital population, which has meant a focus on the confinement of severely schizophrenic patients designated "dangerous to others," who are more often male than female. The overall clinical population, however, is still predominantly female (Horwitz 1982b).

Less is known about mental-hospital life today, ethnographically, than about that of the fifties to early seventies, when most of the pivotal studies were done (Braginsky et al. 1969; Goffman 1961; Perruci 1974). The shift from a more medium or long-term involuntary confinement period to a short-term one would undoubtedly have had an impact on some of the inpatient processes observed by Goffman. For example, the process of "colonization" by which the hospital came gradually to replace the home as the site of self-location and ordinary life is not likely to occur in hospital stays measured in days rather than months, or in weeks rather than years. But other features of the patient career, such as the symptomatization of behavior (the interpretation of all patient behavior by staff as psychiatrically symptomatic), are unlikely to have changed much, considering the relatively unchanged bureaucratic structure of staff—patient relationships (see Lidz et al. 1984).

Since the sixties there has been an additional movement in mental health that has had a profound impact on the lives of persons diagnosed as mentally ill (including some of the Bay Area patients; see follow-up summaries in appendix A): the community mental-health center system. Designed as an alternative to state hospitalization for even chronic schizophrenic patients, these centers provide treatments such as talk and drug therapy on an outpatient basis and also provide various forms of day care. Although there is a vast literature on such centers, it will not be discussed here, since it is not central to the themes of this analysis; suffice it to note that instead of serving the chronic schizophrenics released from the state hospitals, community mental-health centers have tended to be a "net-widening" operation, serving populations previously unserved by psychiatric facilities (Brown 1985). The women in the original study were untouched by this movement, though they were encouraged to undertake outpatient therapy during the year of conditional discharge. In 1972, however, a couple of the women in the follow-up did report using these centers, mainly for the provision of maintenance doses of psychoactive drugs. But most of those followed up were affected by the restriction of state-hospital use, as the epilogue indicates.

THEORIES OF MADNESS

The medicalization of madness and the debate between the organic and psychological etiologists have continued since the fifties. It appears that the somaticists are currently in the ascendant, with genetic and hormonal theories of schizophrenia enjoying considerable popular and scientific support. The specialization characteristic of modern medicine has also continued: the *Diagnostic and Statistical Manual* of the American Psychiatric Association (now DSM III) has subsumed more categories of disorder and used more specific measurements with each succeeding edition.

At the same time, since the fifties there has been a renewed interest in the notion of social organization as the source of madness, rather than the individual's body or family system. Such an approach had some currency in the mid-nineteenth century, when the notion of "moral disorder" replaced the notion of bodily "humors" as the source of mental illness. At that time the cure of moral disorder was moral treatment in the community of the asylum. Today, the social-organization approach to madness takes two forms, one of which involves a profound critique of the asylum.

The premise of this critique is that those very social arrangements designed to effect a cure of mental illness can, and often do, reinforce instead the social role and identity of mental patient (see Goffman 1961; Perruci 1974). The critique of the asylum is one aspect of labeling theory. According to this argument, existing social arrangements create labels such as "mentally ill" or "schizophrenic," which are then used to identify and deal with deviants. At the heart of labeling processes is social control, or the power to make one's labels stick. Labeling theorists have argued that more women receive psychiatric treatment than men because in our society men have more power to control women than vice versa (Horwitz 1982b).

A second social-organization critique focuses on the social structure in general rather than on specific bureaucratic manifestations of it. There has been of late a renewal of interest in both the functionalist and the Marxist critiques of social order as they might be used to explain female madness. For conflict theorists it is the empty wastes of capitalist society that provoke madness; for the functionalists it is—and particularly for women—the strain of social roles. Functionalist anomie or strain theories explain women's depression, neurosis, or other symptoms as a response to the role of women in modern society:

the woman's role in modern industrial societies has a number of characteristics that may promote mental illness. . . . Patterned variations in the rates of mental illness among men and women exist . . . suggesting that the ordering of these rates is a reflection of the position of men and women in society. . . . we need to know much more about how the woman's role produces high rates of mental illness. (Gove and Tudor 1973, 831)

Indeed, since the mid-seventies, a feminist critique of psychiatry has developed the thesis that the history of psychiatry is in many ways a history of the place of women in the social order (see for example, Chodorow 1978; Margolis 1984). Women have been regarded historically as more open to emotional distress than men, from the "vapors" of the nineteenth-century novel heroines to the "imagination" and "spells" of women in the fifties. Previously unquestioned acceptance of such female-discounting psychiatric concepts as "hysteria" and "penis envy" has been replaced by a consciousness of their ideological—and misogynist—character. But the more general and pervasive equation of femaleness with emotionality and unreason has not changed very much (Chesler 1972; Schur 1984; Showalter 1985).

The history of psychiatric treatment and institutionalization has also been reframed as a history of the treatment and institutionalization of women, since more women than men have sought psychiatric treatment and more have been subjected to invasive treatments such as ECT (Gove and Tudor 1973; Horwitz 1982b). And, as I have indicated, scholars have come to recognize the combined authority of psychiatry and the family in the case of both women and children who are mental patients. Although there have been considerable changes in the mental-health system since the fifties—and certainly since the early days of psychiatry—gender remains a powerful shaper and predictor of psychiatric careers. As etiological statements the labeling, functionalist, and feminist conflict theories of female madness are competitive in the sense that they proffer alternative structural explanations. In turn, these sociological theories compete with biological explanations, such as the genetic theory of schizophrenia, and with psychological theories such as that of the "double-binding" family. But if, instead, these sociological theories are taken (reflexively) as historically grounded interpretations that offer sensitizing insights, rather than as ahistorical explanations, then they can be useful. Both the strain of the housewife role and certain labeling or denial practices by husbands (see chapter 6) are implicated in the Bay Area women's experiences of madness. But neither can be seen, simplistically, as causing them. In the next chapter, I will indicate the ways in which the housewife role in the fifties was linked, for these women, to madness.

The Prepatient

CHAPTER 2

Schizophrenic Housewives

The designation of these Bay Area women as mentally ill and in need of hospitalization was made against the background of their marital relationships, which in turn reflected the historical structure of marriage in the 1950s. The original researchers characterized the majority of these marriages (the Bakers, Jameses, Marks, Orens, Prices, Quinns, Rands, Sands, Thornes, Ureys, and Whites) as "separate worlds" characterized by mutual withdrawal:

> The husband often became increasingly involved in his work or in other interests ouside the marital relationship. The wife usually became absorbed in private concerns about herself and her children. . . . The partners . . . achieved a type of marital accommodation based on mutual inaccessibility, emotional distance, and lack of explicit demands on each other. (Sampson et al. 1964, 75)

As Jessie Bernard (1972), Lillian Rubin (1979), and others have shown, separate worlds were not confined to the families of schizophrenics in the era of the Bay Area study, but were typical of traditional marital relationships, especially among the working class. Perhaps less typical was the merged family developed by the Arlens, Karrs, Lows, and Yales, in which "the marital partners and their children did not establish a relatively self-contained nuclear family. Rather, family life was chronically or occasionally organized around the presence of a maternal figure who took over the wife's domestic and child-rearing functions. This person was the wife's mother in three cases, her mother-in-law in the fourth (Arlen)" (Sampson et al. 1964, 83–84). The marital relationships of the

Noons and Vicks were not typologized by the original researchers (for further details on these marriages, see appendix A).

Although the women in the separate-worlds marriages frequently complained about their lack of contact or communication with their husbands, there was no societal discourse available to give form to their dissatisfaction; thus, the expression of dissatisfaction could be—and often was—fed into the developing process of these women's troubles. And since the marriages were not only separate but unequal, the wives were expected to subordinate their concerns to their husbands'. As Peggy Sand said of their marital difficulties: "Oh I've read a lot of books and articles, they all add up to the same thing, baby your husband, build up his ego, all that. I feel that I have one too that needs building up sometimes."

In the fifties, divorce was available and increasing, yet it was not seen as a ready solution to marital difficulties. Although they were dissatisfied, most of the Bay Area spouses—like most of those untouched by hospitalization—continued their marriages even after the Napa episode. But these marriages were, nevertheless, more vulnerable than the average. The Bakers and Quinns were divorced during the period of the original study, while the Thornes were separated and later reconciled. Several of the others had contemplated separation over the years. The original researchers summarized the status of the marriages at the end of the study period; these comments may be compared with table 1.2:

At the time of the last follow-up, seven women were not living in the marital family. Four of the seven (Price, Noon, James and Urey) were in the hospital but still formally married; the objective situation and the psychological status of the marital relationship alike lead us to consider these as instances of unofficial separation. . . . Two of the seven (Vick and Quinn) . . . were living alone in the community; their children were in the care of the husband. The last of the seven (Baker) was living with one child in the community; her other child lived with her former husband. (Sampson et al. 1964, 94)

Patterns of separation and divorce in the Bay Area families were structured by gender. In the case of the Bakers, Quinns, and Thornes it was the husband who left, Mr. Thorne and Mr. Quinn for "the other woman." These men could afford, both economically and emotionally, to desert their families and start new ones. But their wives could not. For women in the fifties the impulse to separation tended to be impotent, because they were not in an economic position to support themselves or their children. The one wife who had left her husband intermittently for more than a decade prior to the study and expressed a wish for divorce in the original study (Peggy Sand) was still married by the 1972 follow-up.

The separateness, inequality, and dissatisfactions of these marriages provided the context for the interpretation and handling of the women's emotional troubles. In the first place, marital troubles became crystallized into those spheres which structured control and dependence: the housewife role, money, sex, and work. Second, personal troubles for the schizophrenic women were experienced as those feelings connected with housewifery: financial dependence and isolation from adult contacts, emotional dependence, depression, feelings of aloneness and abandonment.

Thus, the marital troubles experienced by these couples were patterned in specific ways that reflected themes of control, dominance, and submission as they intersected with the routine tasks of everyday life. His paycheck, her working, his sexual demands, her spending, all provided a context for the interpretation and handling of trouble, and for a schizophrenic diagnosis and hospitalization. In particular, these troubles became entwined in what was probably the most crucial feature of the fifties housewife role: housework.

Trouble and the Housewife Role

It is clear that housework and child care were of central importance to the Bay Area families, not only in the sense of time-consumption and practical activity (the role aspect), but also in the sense of providing a locus for identity (the self aspect) in a structure that provided no alternative sources of female identity.

It is not surprising, then, that much of the trouble in these Bay Area families became crystallized around the housewife role. First, housework and child care can be a source of strain on women, simply by its burdensome, time-consuming, boring, and relentless character. Second, housework can become the repository for male criticism: not doing it well, or on rarer occasions doing it too well, can become a source of insult. Indeed, the women themselves—since their selves were embedded in housework—also engaged in this form of denigration. Finally, the isolation characteristic of traditional housewives who were not integrated into stable kin networks precipitated a sense of trouble and crisis in the lives of married women. All these features of the relations among women, housework, and trouble in the fifties stemmed ultimately from economic powerlessness, something which is not highlighted in the literature on sex roles and mental illness.

As Allan Horwitz notes, the strain of a role is exacerbated by the context of powerlessness within which one is compelled to perform it; "the distress usually attributed to the role of housewives may be more generalizable to the roles of people who occupy subordinate positions" (1982a, 619). He suggests that "deviation from sex-role expectations is productive of distress only when the deviant is lacking in power" (ibid., 620) and concludes that the most stressful situation occurs when the occupant of a powerless role also deviates from sex-appropriate behavior (ibid., 607). This complex of factors well describes the situation of the Bay Area women. A parodic example was provided by Ruth Quinn, who, prior to mental hospitalization had been physically ill and unable to do her housework. (This and subsequent passages are cited from the unpublished transcripts of interviews with the Bay Area families and researchers' reports.) "After visiting her doctor: Mrs. Quinn . . . told me about the note which she got from Dr. M. and which she had intended to give to her husband . . . stating that she has a bladder infection and this is why she isn't able to do her housework."

In the fifties, women were expected to find self-fulfillment in housework and child care, to work outside the home (if they had young children) only if it was financially necessary, and to regard housework as a challenging career. Those women who did not wholeheartedly endorse this program—which included all the Bay Area women at least some of the time—were viewed as at least troublesome, if not unfeminine, and perhaps in the extreme case crazy. Thus, the strain inherent in the role of the powerless housewife went unrecognized, except perhaps latently, by the original scholarly analysts and from time to time by some of the Bay Area wives and husbands themselves. Among the Bay Area women, the most clearly dissatisfied wife, with the most clearly articulated sense of protest, was Kate White; even she, however, was ambivalent about whether to interpret her feelings and ambitions by prevailing cultural norms or by her own reasoning processes:

She felt that in many ways she did not have the same goals and ideas as her neighborhood. This awakened in her the old conflict she had talked about in the past about whether she had to conform or not and whether not conforming meant that something was wrong with her. In the past she had felt that all her nonconformist behavior, all her rebellion, were signs of mental illness. Now she didn't think this was necessarily so.

Because of the central significance of housework in the traditional housewife role, having trouble with chores was troublesome to both wives and husbands. To wives, nonperformance of tasks meant they were incompetent, both in their own eyes and the eyes of others; if this sense of incompetence became too extreme, it could be and was interpreted as part of a descent into madness. The husbands, by contrast, interpreted incompetence at housework as troublesome primarily from the vantage point of getting things conveniently accomplished. A wife who did not do the dishes or get the children off to school was, in the fifties, no wife at all.

Although both husbands and wives spoke of housework as a source of those troubles that led up to hospitalization, for the wife it was a cause of trouble—the demands of the role provoked stress—while for the husband it was a symptom—the failure to perform it adequately. Jack Oren, for example, equated "flipping out" with the inability to perform housework: "She flipped, that's all, how else would you put it, baby couldn't play outside, doors were all locked, when I say flipped, she wasn't well enough to take care of the house." Similarly, when asked how his wife's troubles had started, Tim Quinn said, "She wouldn't get out of bed and wouldn't do a doggone thing, and became as lethargic as an alligator in the sun" (a comment that, even in the fifties, the hospital thought worthy of inclusion in Mrs. Quinn's admission files). Although in almost all cases it was undone or incomplete housework that signaled trouble, in a few instances it was overenthusiastic role performance: "*Mel Noon:* I asked Mr Noon when he first started wondering that his wife might be mentally sick. He said, 'I started wondering—she was cleaning up the house ten times a day—immaculate, didn't have to be.'"

While inadequate housework was a trouble symptom to the husbands, to the wives themselves it was also a cause. Many of the wives traced their troubles to the demands of the housewife role, including housework. Donna Urey, for example, commented:

"how I got this way—I had five children very close together . . . with young children so close together, a wife and a husband disagree because a certain amount of housework isn't done—and the wife is very emotionally upset due to the fact that she knows she has too many duties to perform, and therefore she finds it is overwhelming and one has so many children to take care of in this day and age, and of course young children are quite a load on a lot of people's shoulders. . . . I was feeling upset during . . . the time that I was in the midst of my pregnancy with the twins . . . there was a lot of misguided feelings that I had within myself . . . I started hearing these delusions. . . . I was very neat up to that time I had the second child, and after that everything seemed to go from the neatness to the sloppiness. . . . We didn't have time to really sit down and relax. We didn't have enough time to be together as husband and wife . . . I didn't have time enough for the children and everything seemed to be in one big turmoil and that's how I felt."

Taking care of children was, as Donna Urey commented, another stressful aspect of the housewife role. And the more children, the more difficulties. In our culture, even more perhaps in the fifties than today, motherhood is romanticized and glorified, though it remains economically unrewarded and pragmatically unsupported. It may be because of this cultural ideology that, in contrast to their willingness to express discontent with housework, the Bay Area women were reluctant to trace any of their troubles to the strain of caring for their children.

Both the Bay Area women and their husbands, however, linked the women's emotional distress to hormonal changes attendant upon childbirth. Many of the women traced the origins of their difficulties to the birth of one or more children, and several of them were diagnosed as suffering from "post-partum depression" as well as schizophrenia. The husbands, too, turned to this culturally legitimated explanation:

Leo Vick: He attributed his wife's hospitalization to her being "nervous" because she had had measles, they had moved a lot, and the birth of her third child.

Jack Oren: "Right after the baby's birth her breasts rose up and she had pain and couldn't sleep." He added that he had been told that "a year or two after the birth of a baby something like this happens—routine." I asked him who told him this and he said "told this by . . . gynecologist . . . year or so after you have a baby, sometimes crack a bit."

The tasks of housework and child care were undertaken by these women in isolation from adult company, at least in those families not integrated into stable kin networks. Donna Urey expressed her sense of isolation as a housewife, in addition to the burden of housework and caring for five children:

[she heard] "voices like guardian angels [who] steered me away from distrust of my husband . . . he would be downstairs working, and I'd think, 'gee willikers, why doesn't he come up to have a cup of coffee' because he usually did when he first started working on the car, so I'd get upset. 'Cause I'd be ironing and that I—mostly I think it was because I was lonely for him—because even now he says when he leaves me alone he's downstairs and

I'm upstairs. It's like when he leaves for his day's work. I'm left at home by myself with the day's work. We're fine on the weekend because we're together and working like a team. When he leaves and I'm alone and after that I get all confused—I feel alone. I have that alone feeling, and I think that's where it all stems from."

As Joyce Noon commented about her hospitalization: "They all keep telling me that all I needed was tranquilizers [laughs]. Really what I would like to have is someone to stay with us."

Isolation was part of the traditional housewife role, with its solitary tasks and emotional dependence on an absent husband. To be both dependent and isolated made for feelings of abandonment, loneliness, and fear of being left alone, especially in those families characterized by mutual withdrawal. Kate White said:

Like when Josie [daughter] was born, my husband was working eight hours a day and going to school at night. Then he decided to fly on weekends. I never saw him. I didn't feel like a wife or have any feeling about having anything to do with a family. I guess I was a nervous mother at that time too. Josie had the colic and I didn't seem to be able to do anything right. I objected to my husband's [working] on weekends, even though the money was somewhat handy. He said that I was being too possessive . . . I told him I wasn't possessive, and then we would get into an argument. . . . I guess I want too much . . . I guess I wanted my husband to show me things and to reflect reality for me.

And Donna Urey, when asked if there was anything that upset her besides the housework and child care, said, "Well . . . when my husband left . . . everybody says, 'well, how can you get lonesome when you have five children?' I said, 'well I like to talk to a grown-up once in a while.'"

Their lack of contact with the outside world, together with their emotional dependence on their husbands, engendered a sense of alienation from reality and from self. In a very real sense many of these women experienced marital powerlessness as a detachment from life itself, as if they had shifted the burden of experiencing self and world onto their husbands' shoulders. The husbands' resentment at such a maneuver, in view of the situation, was quite as "natural" as the wives' attempting it:

Mrs. White talked about her husband's lack of effectively reflecting reality for her. Also, he didn't react to her. This meant both that he didn't respond and also that he didn't accept what her feelings were on any particular issue. "Like when we settle down—he came home with the idea of going overseas. I said it was impossible, he couldn't do it. But later he kept coming home and mentioning it. I got so I felt that maybe I shouldn't feel the way I felt."

The paradox of the "separate worlds" marriage was for the wife a situation of extreme emotional dependence on a husband who was often literally not there, and who was metaphorically "not there" as a provider of intimate communication. The separation problem was even more difficult for these women: Ruth Quinn's feelings of isolation were heightened by her husband's desertion, especially at the times he used to provide company for her. "I do very well during the day—which is natural, since the children and Tim were always gone during the day. It's around dinner time that I feel lonely. Last night I felt a little around that time—I cooked my dinner and listened to the radio. But just around that dinner hour, it's hard."

The husbands' interviews are filled with examples of their wives' clinging to them in a literal or metaphorical sense, behavior that they claimed not to understand at all (at least until the crisis of hospitalization). Some of the wives tried to keep their husbands "in sight" as much as possible, following them from room to room or trying to prevent them from going to work. In the course of explaining a fire that occurred one day as he was leaving for work, Arnold Baker said, "I don't know how the fire got started, she was at the window. . . . When I'm outside she's at the window all the time, looking at me." The isolation experienced by Mrs. Baker was reflected in the trouble she caused her neighbors, which became part of her mental illness. Mr. Baker describes it:

"she was walking into the neighbors' houses all the time without knocking, and they didn't like it. You wouldn't like it either." [In a later episode] "The night before . . . I took her back to the hospital she went over to the neighbor's across the street and was on their porch. The fellow came out and said to her, 'now go home or you'll go back to Napa.'" (What was she doing over there?) "I don't know. I guess she went into other people's houses or onto the porch because she was trying to find somebody to talk to."

PSYCHIATRIC SYMPTOMS AND THE HOUSEWIFE

The problems in everyday living experienced by these women—loneliness, isolation, and the stress of the housewife role—were reflections of the conventional structure of marriage and family in the fifties. But they were also psychiatric symptoms. A careful analysis of these women's communications reveals the ways in which their delusions and hallucinations were metaphors for their social place (for another example, see Schatzman 1975). Eve Low, for example, saw herself as having been hypnotized by her husband and her doctors, as punished for her offenses by ECT, and as the victim of a master conspiracy to rob her of control of her own life. A psychiatrist said she had: "a very complicated set of delusions . . . that she is . . . the legitimate or illegitimate daughter of some people, and in an attempt to deny her these rights there are conspirators who have managed to get her put in the state hospital."

In reality, Eve Low had been coerced into hospitalization by a coalition of marital and psychiatric authority, forced into ECT against her will, and inducted into a total institution in which her life was regulated by others (Goffman 1961). Eve Low and two other patients also expressed delusional beliefs that they were someone else, or that they were married to someone else. Such a claim detaches the patient from the family context entirely, removing her metaphorically from the source of her distress: "Eve Low said that all her life she believed she was Ellen Lamb. When she was married it was under that name. However, since she has recently discovered that she is really Lily Barnes, she believes that the marriage may not be legal and she may no longer be married."

Donna Urey's case history can be read, similarly, as the history of a housewife. Donna Urey—who had resorted to a number of quite ordinary strategies for keeping her husband or children in the house as company for her—also heard voices. Whatever the other features of these voices, they provided human sounds in an empty environment. She says, furthermore, that these voices "steered her away" from paranoid delusions about her husband, and that she heard voices "mostly I think it was because I was lonely." Joyce Noon's delusions, too, might be interpreted as metaphors for gender relations within the traditional family. She said that she "imagined" that "there was an apartment over her mother's house where a husband and wife lived. 'I argued with him all the time, mostly with him, because he wouldn't let her talk.'"

The two women most overtly at odds with the traditional housewife role—Kate White and Mary Yale—both had delusions about homosexuality and (in Mary's case) about turning into a man (see also Messinger and Warren 1984). Mr. Yale implied a latent awareness of psychiatric metaphor when he said of his wife's involvement with the woman upstairs (whom Mary had accused of being a "homosexual"): "I was paying too much attention to my friends and too little to her. . . . She began to take a very deep interest in the lady upstairs." Thus the delusion of "homosexuality" in the "lady upstairs" substituted for a sense of closeness and communication with Mary's husband.

But while the role of housewife was a source of emotional distress to the Bay Area women, it nevertheless provided a sense of place. To be a wife and mother was the only fully legitimate social place, in fact, open to the fifties woman. Indeed, those madwives whose fantasies led them to contemplate separation, or who looked back with nostalgia to their premarriage days (see chapter 4), were held in place ideologically by the metaphor of "old maid," just as they were held in place economically by personal indigence. Whenever the women contemplated being alone, they tempered perception of the benefits of release from an unsatisfactory marriage with the pariah status of the old maid.

Furthermore, the impending loss of their place as housewives was, for Joan Baker, Cora Thorne, and Ruth Quinn, enough to precipitate extreme distress. Joan Baker, who had often imagined separation from a husband who "rejected and depreciated" her (Sampson et al. 1964, 134), became frightened and threatened violence toward her family when Arnold left her for another woman (ibid., 135). Ruth Quinn, whose husband constantly criticized her for excessive weight and faulty housework, was hospitalized shortly after Tim Quinn revealed his intention—expressed and acted upon several prior times—to leave her (see the epilogue). Both Ruth Quinn and Cora Thorne, whose husband left her for another woman, attempted suicide in the face of their husbands' rejection of them.

The threatened loss of the marital relationship was also important in the psychiatric careers of Kate White and Mary Yale. Mary Yale, who felt caught between the emotional demands of her mother and her husband, finally came to the realization that she would lose George if she did not resolve what had become a triadic situation. Although the Yales were hopeful about the future of their marriage immediately following Mary's release from Napa, they separated and reconciled several times during the period of the original study and were again separated at the time of the 1972 follow-up (see the epilogue). The Whites's marriage was intact—at least from Nelson White's point of view—prior to Kate's hospitalization. At the last interview in 1961, however, "Mrs. White was on leave from the state hospital [and] her husband was having an extramarital affair with his secretary." (ibid., 164).

Money, Sex, and Trouble

In return for the performance of household duties, the fifties wife expected financial support for herself and her children. John Clausen and Marian Yarrow (1955), Charlotte Schwartz (1957), and others have documented the ways wives defined their husbands' behavior as troubled when it seems to indicate inadequate performance of the provider role, and the way they try to deny trouble if the provider role is adequately performed. As Schwartz notes, "A wife may place little emphasis on her husband's 'strange ideas' if he demonstrates that he can fulfill the roles of wager earner, husband, and father" (1957, 289).

According to the division of labor in the Bay Area families, like those of the working-class families studied by Lillian Rubin (1976), the wives were responsible for the distribution and allotment of family finances. One of the loci of trouble as perceived by the Bay Area husbands was in the wives' "inordinate" financial demands and "frivolous" spending. As Floyd Sand said, " 'There's always friction between us, it's mostly over the money situation—that's all, it started out the day I married her. I'd get a little nest egg put away, she'd spend it.' . . . He complained that his wife 'Doesn't know the value of a dollar, doesn't look at price when she buys something, whether or not we could afford it.'"

The husbands did not change the division of labor permanently to take over this task in response to the repeated troubles these wives were seen as having at keeping to their budgets, though some did so sporadically. In her comparison of middle- and working-class families, Rubin explains this apparent paradox in the context of discretionary income:

Observers of American family life often point to the fact that so many women handle the family finances as evidence that they wield a great deal of power and influence in the family [three-quarters of Rubin's working-class sample of fifty]. A look behind that bare fact, however, suggests some other conclusions. Among the professional middle-class families, for example, where median income is $22,000 (among the working class it is $12,300)— a level that allows for substantial discretionary spending—the figures flip over almost perfectly; the men manage the money in three-quarters of the families. Moreover, among those working class families where some discretion in spending exists, almost always the husband handles the money, or the wife pays the bills while he makes the decisions (1976, 107).

Her handling the money permits the husbands "to avoid confronting the painful reality that they are not bringing home enough money to buy all the necessities they need and the comforts they would like. If he hands over his pay check and it doesn't quite stretch far enough, he can behave as if the problem lies not with his inadequate income but with her shortcomings as a manager" (ibid., 109).

It is clear that the Bay Area husbands saw their wives' fiscal behavior as troublesome, but they did not see it as one of the symptoms of their wives' diagnosed schizophrenia. I found no instances in which the subjects of the study considered fiscal extravagance as a symptom of mental illness. Indeed, a number of these husbands displayed some awareness that their wives' mental troubles might in some way be related to their sense of inadequacy and powerlessness in the face of inadequate income and lack of control over the provider role. For their part, the wives seemed to sense that their payoffs in the marital bargain were unequal, just as their outlay (in housework) was excessive. They exchanged control over the consumption of income and the withholding of sexual relations for control over the earning of income.

The Sands provided a typical example of the marital bargain in their location of marital trouble. Mr. Sand described their marital difficulties as follows:

I then asked him if he thought there was anything wrong with his wife. "Well . . . I've been with her twelve years—stayed in debt all the time— get $300 ahead, she'd get the bank book—have any bonds, she'd cash 'em." He complained more about how his wife would just spend money, not make any account of it. He would then question her about it, and she would clam up—"Then she wonders why I blow my stack."

Mrs. Sand located the source of their marital troubles in Mr. Sand's excessive sexual demands. She said:

"I can't talk to my husband—I'm afraid of him. . . . My husband is very demanding sexually, he wants to go all the time." . . . She said that when she would not have relations so often, "he would accuse me of playing with myself, or getting it on the side," that otherwise he wouldn't see how Peggy would do without it for so long. Her husband would say about her "there's something wrong with me."

Each told anecdotes that illustrated, within her or his separate interpretive framework, specifically troublesome incidents:

He said that a couple of months ago his wife had bought for the kids a stamp collecting book and a lot of stamps. "Then, all of a sudden, she wrote about every stamp agent in the country. Then . . . she just went overboard, she knows I couldn't pay for all of that."

I then asked her if they had sexual relations while she was home. She answered, "Once, not by agreement, first place, having my menstrual period, he woke up Sunday night. He insisted. He woke me up, I just can't resist with him." I then said to her that she hadn't wanted to, and she shook her head. "No, he kept saying he wanted to love me—I guess that's all he means by love."

In the structure of the working-class marital relationship, the husband is perceived as in control of the sexual aspect of marriage; it is he who requires, and initiates, intercourse (Rubin 1976). Conversely, the woman is dependent on the husband's initiation of sexual activities and on his actions as a source of gratification. Men are seen as physiologically dependent on sexual gratification and females as more in control of their sexual desires. As Rubin says, "historically, it is men, not women, whose sexuality has been thought to be unruly and ungovernable—destined to be restrained by a good (read, asexual) woman" (ibid., 136).

In the fifties, the need for pleasure in sex, and the drive toward fulfillment, were seen even more than in the seventies (when Rubin did her research) as predominantly male characteristics. Women were viewed as receptacles and need-fulfillers, and often as reluctant ones. Shirley Arlen said of the couple's sexual difficulties that " 'I think it was all my fault that I just . . . didn't want to.' She read in the *Readers Digest* that 'once a husband gets this sex drive that it's hard to control it' and that 'you should build up your husband's confidence in himself and tell him that he's . . . a good lover.' "

The Bay Area respondents' sexual problems were related not only to sexual socialization in the fifties family, but also to the prevailing state of contraceptive and abortion technology, legislation, and ideology. Not only those Bay Area couples who were Catholic but also some of those who were not—like the Arlens—opposed contraception, while abortion was legally unavailable. Thus, these men and women sometimes had "unplanned" children and sometimes avoided sexual relations in order not to have them: neither adaptation was particularly beneficial to the marital relationship. In the Arlens' marriage, for example, she blamed their sexual problems not only on her lack of desire but also on the problem of unwanted pregnancy—difficulties that might not have been unrelated. She commented, "I just wish that I could have a correct way to prevent having children so I could make love freely and satisfy my husband, live happily, and just relax. . . . I would so much like to be able to make love with my husband and just have no problems there."

Sexuality and its use as a weapon in traditional marriage was understood by these women, at least implicitly, as the obverse of the economic domination that shaped their lives. Sexual withholding or "inordinate" sexual demands, extramarital affairs or homosexual "delusions" appeared as manifestations of trouble among them, in addition to "overspending" or doing an "inadequate" job at housework. It is hardly surprising, therefore, that sexual interaction was a significant arena, in a number of the marital dyads, in which trouble was located and defined.

The husbands generally concurred in their wives' self-blame for sexual difficulties. Their complaints about their wives' sexual response centered around two opposing sorts of trouble: withdrawal of sexual contact or responsiveness, and excessive or "peculiar" sexual demands. The husbands did not regard their wives' sexual withdrawal or lack of response as a sign of abnormality, since this fitted into the established paradigm of male and female control and dependence in the sexual area. In the working-class marriage in general, "he asks; she gives. And neither is satisfied with the resolution" (Rubin 1976, 136). However, if excessive sexuality was the trouble, then the paradigm was violated, and such behavior could easily be perceived as a symptom of mental illness. Extramarital liaisons with other men provided particular evidence of craziness, since affairs were considered a paradigmatically male, not female, type of "normal trouble." After Joyce Noon's release, Mel Noon had his wife returned to the hospital after he had found her in a bar very late at night, talking to a man, having left their son at home:

"The last time I sent her to Napa I sent her good and fast that time . . . I was so mad as hell . . . I grabbed her by the throat and started choking and I choked her as hard as I could squeeze. I would have killed her if I hadn't stopped when I did . . . I said . . . I give you a choice. Either you go to the hospital tomorrow morning or I'll call the police and have them take you back."

Almost the identical course of action was pursued by Mr. Sand when he discovered that his wife was having an affair with a fellow patient while at Napa.

Although the wives did not generally define their sexual troubles as a response to their difficulties with the traditional structure of marriage, it is at least a reasonable hypothesis that a number of them used sex to protest the inequality in their marriages. It is clear that these wives' sexual troubles were explicable sociologically, as instances of their troubled lives and marriages in general, not just psychiatrically, as symptoms reflecting their depression and mental disorder.

WORK OUTSIDE THE HOME

Some of the Bay Area women held jobs prior to marriage or childbearing: two were photojournalists, two elementary school teachers, one was a waitress, one a secretary, and one a theater usherette. They were typical of the women of the fifties in that all of them gave up working either as soon as they got married or when they had their first child. By the time of the Bay Area interviews, the issue of work outside the home had become a source of trouble in these women's marital relationships. One aspect of the provider role for the lower- to middle-class male in the fifties was that, to seem successful, he must be the sole supporter of the entire family. On the one hand, wives who worked symbolized inadequacy and role failure. On the other, the financial condition of the lower- to lower-middle-class families, exacerbated sometimes by the wives' spending habits, was rather perilous, and there was a felt need for the wives to work. In either case, the control over the decision whether the wives would work rested ultimately in the husband, not in the wife.

In light of these circumstances, it is not surprising that the stance of most of the husbands toward their wives' working might be described as ambivalent, fluctuating between reluctant approval and unrealistic disapproval. The wives seemed overtly to accept the division of labor in the family whereby the husbands made the ultimate decision about wives' work. The use of the phrases "he won't let me work" or "if he lets me work" was a common expression of their lack of control. Joyce Noon:

I mean I might go to work but that wouldn't be any good because we don't need the money. It might do me some good to work but he just isn't giving in, that's all, and he never will. I might as well be sitting up here [at Napa] as doing anything else because I'm never going to get past him. But he is just not ever giving up. . . . So I'm just as well off up here. . . . I can't go to work, he won't let me go to work. I'm all right when I stay home but I get tired of staying alone.

Nevertheless, there was a considerable amount of covert struggle over the issue. The women who wanted to work expressed a great deal of resentment over their powerlessness:

Interviewer: "When the three of us met, you referred to male chauvinism. What did you mean?"
Kate White: "Oh, Mr. White maintains he has no male chauvinism at all, yet I do think so. Often when he comes home he's kind of condescending about my staying home and doing the housework. On the one hand he talks of money, and that we can't plan ahead on the money he makes—but as though he were reconciled to the fact that it's perfectly OK for me to stay at home because I'm a woman anyway."

Although the troubles caused by wives in the areas of overspending and withdrawal from sexual activities were not readily attributed to mental illness, since they fitted the paradigm of the female role, being sexually demanding was more readily perceived as a symptom of psychiatric trouble. And the will to work in a way that would wrest control of the process from the husbands was ouside the paradigm, and therefore liable to be seen as mad. Kate White was perceived as "crazy" in part because of her desire to be a "career woman," something that was an "inexplicable" rejection of the feminine role.

In Kate White's case, the concept of craziness became mixed up ineluctably with the concept of work and career. She talked about getting a job, but her husband was adamantly opposed to it. His negative views were reinforced by other relatives; Kate's aunt "lectured" her against being a "career woman." But for Kate herself, the "housewife and diaper routine" was in itself a source of "craziness"; she attributed recurrent feelings of "going crazy" to her housewife-and-mother role, while her husband and aunt attributed craziness to her career ambitions. Peggy Sand also located the deep source of her troubles in the economic structure of her marriage: "I asked if there was anything else involved in her husband not wanting her to work. 'I don't know.' And after a pause, added 'might be he wants to keep me dependent on him for money—he probably does.'"

There were—and are—reasons for work not functioning as a panacea for troubled housewives in the fifties. The women who had worked were aware of the twin problems associated with simultaneous housework and outside work: the fact that women thus do two rather than one job, and the limited quality of work available to most women. Eve Low, who had earlier attempted to combine housewifery with elementary-school teaching, commented, "It's difficult. If you work days. You come home and you have to get dinner and get the children settled and iron a dress and go to bed and get up and do the same thing—but if it's the only way that I'm going to be able to have anything and have any kind of secure existence at all I guess I have to do it." In comparing the lives of housewives and of office workers, Joyce Noon found both wanting:

I used to work in an office and everybody treated the poor private secretary like an outcast—she's usually an old maid and you know how they are. . . .

Wives, housewives and mothers are peculiar. Nobody ever bothers them because nobody wants to do what they are doing. . . . Office workers get no appreciation. Usually they're joining clubs and awful picky and poking, lonely and grouchy, I don't know.

There is no doubt, however, that the idea of work did represent a fantasized way out of their financial and emotional troubles for many of the Bay Area women. The reality might be that work would be onerous and boring; the dream was that it would provide an escape from isolation and drudgery. Indeed, the literature on housewives who work outside the home does indicate that work, despite its limitations and added burdens, functions for women in just these ways (Margolis 1984). During her hospitalization, for example, Donna Urey applied for a job as a magazine writer, planning to divorce her husband and escape the demands of her five children.

Going to work was one way the Bay Area women proposed to achieve economic and personal (and sometimes marital) independence; conversely, economic dependence was a major factor inhibiting the desire of some of these women for separation from their husbands. As Joan Baker said, she was worried about the future of her marriage and whether she wanted it or not, but "I have never gone out to support myself—that's a hell of a reason for staying, I know, just because he supports me."

Two of the Bay Area women did get jobs during the period of marital change and readjustment that followed hospitalization. Shirley Arlen, who had never worked before, applied for a department-store job without mentioning her Napa stay and obtained it; over the next few years she had several similar jobs. She repeated many times during the interviews that she "feels fine" when working but not during her "laid off" periods. Though trained and previously employed as a photojournalist, Mary Yale found a job as a waitress following hospitalization. This step was taken in the face of her husband's antagonism; he said she was too "nervous" to work.

While complaining of marital difficulties, the Bay Area women did not themselves make the analysis of their situation that I made in chapter

1. They were lonely, isolated, dissatisfied, and depressed, but they did not link these and other life problems with the economic dependence and submission that characterized the gender role of the fifties wife. One woman, not in the sample but observed by a researcher at her discharge conference, did come close to recognizing the structural determinants of her difficulties, expressing a resubmission to the demands of housewifery:

> *Staff member:* "What had brought this on? . . . Why did you come in?"
> *Lily Nixon:* "I was advised to."
> *Staff:* "Why?"
> *Lily Nixon:* "I felt I was dominated."
> *Staff:* "By your husband?"
> *Lily Nixon:* "Yes . . . I felt that I was dominated. Now, I've had a chance to think things out."

The social situation of the housewife formed the background to the crisis of schizophrenia and hospitalization, but it was not the sole cause of the crisis. In most cases, even in the fifties, it took more than inadequate role performance for husbands to commit wives involuntarily to the mental hospital, and it took more than the strain of housewifery for women to admit themselves. In the next chapter, I examine some of the ways in which being a woman and a housewife in the fifties combined with other experiences to precipitate the crisis of hospitalization.

CHAPTER 3

The Crisis of Hospitalization

Hospitalization at Napa crystallized prior troubles into psychiatric form. During the first days and weeks of hospitalization, the Bay Area respondents developed theories of why the trouble had come about, what were its origins, and what the future held. For all the families, the troubles that preceded hospitalization had had a long history, either of the wife's bizarre behavior and the husband's attempts to cope with it, or of the wife's feelings of distress and the husband's awareness. Trouble must be noticed before it can be interpreted and remedied.

The natural history of these women's troubles in a sense began with hospitalization, since hospitalization prompted them to restructure their biographies as those of mental patients. Such a dramatic event as hospitalization requires, in our culture, some explanation; in the Bay Area study, furthermore, the interviews were designed to elicit accounts of how and why it happened. Thus the natural history of trouble and its remedies is on its surface a history of the past; but in a more fundamental sense it is a history of the present (Smith 1978; 1983).

For the Bay Area families, the process of accounting for the pre-patient's troubles took the form of a search for the situational (immediate) and the deeper causes of the wife's newly diagnosed schizophrenia. In the first days and weeks of hospitalization the wives and husbands began the process of examining and reshaping biography. This process took place within a particular interpretive context: the medical model. As Jaber Gubrium and David Buckholdt note, the introduction of professional expertise into biographical reinterpretation is significant (1977). Professionals tend to make people's lives seem more coherent and ordered than they would otherwise:

A variety of professionals claim to have special expertise in discovering individual biographies. . . . Not having a publicly codified technology of doing biographical work suggests that the latitude and tolerance of typifications among lay persons are wider and higher, respectively, than among professionals. A biography generated by a professional is more likely to have stylized patterning than one generated by a lay person. Patterning and stylization aside, however, all people engage in the practical work that categorizes behavior displays as one type of conduct or another. The difference between lay and professional biographers lies not in their practice but in the stock of knowledge by which each interprets past lives. (ibid., 168)

Thus, the Bay Area respondents learned to combine everyday and psychiatric interpretations in their accounts of what happened to the pre-patient; as I will elaborate in chapter 7, this process continued in the ex-patient stage.

Biographies and autobiographies also differ from each other: in their coherence, stylization, stock of knowledge, and perspective. Coherence and stylization are derived not only from an external, professional stock of knowledge, but also from an absence of firsthand experience. The Napa psychiatrists had little understanding of their patients' everyday lives, while the husbands were routine observers. But only the wives experienced their troubles and felt their own distress. Thus, the husbands' accounts of their wives' difficulties were at once more coherent and more open to psychiatric interpretation than their wives'. The two accounts of what happened and why diverged considerably, not necessarily because one or another of the spouses was a liar, but because they did not, in the end, share the world they seemed to share.

A Natural History of Trouble

The natural history of these women's troubles began with the awareness of trouble and ended with the crisis of hospitalization. Following the failure of lesser remedial attempts, the last resort of hospitalization precipitated the women into patienthood. And from the moment they were labeled as schizophrenic, the process of accounting for this crisis began. The nature of the cues that signaled trouble, the response to difficulties, the trouble theories developed, and the remedial steps attempted were all shaped by the gender dynamics of the fifties family.

The process of becoming troubled involves both subjective and interpersonal elements. Those Bay Area women who were isolated from their spouses and others in their married lives and who admitted themselves to the hospital had undergone a process (of whatever length) of increasing dissatisfaction with their relationships and of internal emotional trouble that had not been shared with or noticed by their uninvolved husbands. Some of these "separate-worlds" wives had been committed by thier husbands following a "last-straw" incident (of which more later) in which they had forcibly brought their difficulties to the attention of their spouses. Others had simply dealt with their own troubles by seeking admission to Napa.

The husbands became aware of their wives' troubles in a number of different ways. Six of the husbands said in the initial interviews that they didn't notice anything was wrong with their wives until just prior to—in some cases the day of—hospitalization. Mr. Karr said, "if her mother never called up—I wouldn't have known till I went down to see her [at the hospital]." Mr. Low: "I guess I was too darn busy trying to make a living that I didn't pay to much attention to it." Mr. Thorne: "the neighbors would just kind of keep it to themselves and I guess they figured I knew what was going on—I didn't." Mr. Oren: "I didn't notice too much—but the neighbors did." Furthermore, six of the husbands reported that others defined the condition as psychiatric before they did, despite the fact that most of the women's lives were spent in the home, with the husband more often present than anyone except the children. As Mr. Price summarized, "I didn't realize she was out of her head."

Other studies indicate gender differences in spouses' awareness of emotional troubles. In interviews with the wives of male mental patients during the fifties, researchers who asked these women what went wrong prior to hospitalization did not report an unawareness response (compare Yarrow et al. 1955 with Warren 1983). In the context of the traditional marital relationship, it is not surprising that wives notice more about their husbands' state of mind than husbands do about their wives'. Noticing the emotions of others is part of women's traditional emotional labor. And for the fifties wives, quite literally their well-being—both financial and emotional—depended on their husbands. The opposite was not true. Therefore, the stakes for monitoring the spouses' emotional well-being were high for wives, and not for husbands. Female socialization, in the context of dependence and control, teaches women to notice; male socialization, in the context of a lack of reciprocity, teaches them to overlook.

What was noticed as troublesome varied with the individual and with the couple. The women, with access to their inner feelings and thoughts, became aware of their own distress and of its effect on the conduct of their everyday lives as housewives and mothers. Some husbands, with access only to their wives' communications and behavior, sometimes noticed nothing and sometimes only noticed dramatic "last straws." But other husbands, as I discussed in the previous chapter, reported that they had observed a series of untoward actions and communications for a period of time prior to hospitalization, ranging from violations of the housewife role to delusions and hallucinations.

DELUSIONS AND HALLUCINATIONS

Among the classic psychiatric symptoms of schizophrenia are hallucinations or bizarre delusions: seeing, hearing, or believing things that have only internal reality. Among the Bay Area women, Donna Urey,

Kate White, and Joyce Noon heard voices, while Kate White, Mary Yale, Eve Low, Irene James, Wanda Karr, June Mark, Rose Price, Ann Rand, and Cora Thorne were delusional. These women's delusions revolved around their social place: they were someone else, they were married to someone else, they were being persecuted by neighbors or by the CIA.

The husbands whose wives had been hallucinating or delusional for some time came to that conclusion gradually, proposing and discarding alternative explanations for strange actions and statements (Warren 1983; Yarrow et al. 1955): "Mr. White: At Easter time she became quite religious and it was quite obvious that she was becoming disturbed. She began to comment on messages coming from planes, parked cars . . . she went to the church and gave up her wedding ring . . . she had two husbands (she said), Mr. White and her psychiatrist."

The process of identifying communications as delusional was affected both by general cultural notions of plausibility and by the nomic character of the marital relationship. Delusions sometimes met the edge of plausibility without going over it, referring to behavior or actions on the part of others that would seem unlikely but not impossible. In the prepatient stage, husbands often accepted such beliefs as real rather than delusional. Borderline events or pseudoevents were readily considered believable:

Mr. White: He felt his wife misinterpreted a good deal of what [her outpatient psychiatrist] told her. She had told him [husband] that Dr. J had shouted at her and searched her purse the first time she entered his office. "I guess that could be. He might suspect she was a dope addict, but then a doctor could usually recognize this without having to search the purse. Besides, I'm sure it would be unlikely for a dope addict to carry the stuff in her purse."

The boundaries of plausibility are far more plastic in the marital context—especially in an enduring marriage—than in a less intimate relationship (Horwitz 1982b; Warren 1983; Yarrow et al. 1955). For the nonintimate observer, delusions stretch the boundaries of belief to the breaking point when they refer to the conspiratorial behavior of inanimate objects, such as persecution by rays from a TV set. And yet marital relations have been observed to accommodate such beliefs within their everyday fabric (Yarrow et al. 1955). It is perhaps because of the obdurate character of everyday life, and of marriage as the firmest of dyadic lifeworlds (Berger and Kellner 1970), that implausibilities can be entertained as plausibilities. Occasionally, in the prehospital stage, husbands believed what most cultural actors would regard as implausible versions of events. Mr. Yale, for example, "said he had half-believed her delusions about . . . turning into a man." Albert Urey explained his prepatient interpretations of his wife's delusions:

"We'd moved into this old house. I was working late hours. My wife couldn't sleep at night. There was an attic there. The house made noises, the way old houses do. She was frightened, she used to think there was someone in the house with the kids." (What did you think?) "The way the house was situated, old and creaky, a person can think a lotta things."

He talked about the voices his wife heard:

"what I attributed it to is the way the house was set. It was set back, and the street was fairly busy. And people were walking by, their voices would echo in, and I mean that's why I didn't think anything of it, I mean I just thought it was her imagination. If I heard her talking, I mean, I don't think anything of anybody talking to themselves, I do it myself sometimes. . . . but this was definitely—I mean because after I first heard it, well then I'd listen to what was going on, and she was actually arguing with whoever was there—whoever she thought was there."

Similarly, Paul Mark took as real events what he later came to define as hallucinations. "She thought Indians were coming after her. I checked the [nearby drive-in] movie, and they had a Western with Indians in it that night. She also thought that hot rodders were coming after me. I think she heard a motor running outside." Mr. Mark's "checking" of the

drive-in movie indicates the routine ways in which the Bay Area husbands attempted to cope with their wives' delusions.

As Robert Emerson and Sheldon Messinger point out, initial attempts to remedy delusional behavior are intrinsic in character; that is,
attempts are made directly to change the behavior seen as problematic
(1977). While Mr. Mark checked the drive-in movie—implicitly believing his wife's story—Mr. Urey attempted to alleviate Donna Urey's fear of
the attic in their house by persuasion and example. As Mrs. Urey reports:

[Our old house] had an attic, and that scared the life out of me because I
wasn't used to an attic. It seems funny, doesn't it? It had a great big attic
inside of the closet. That's how it all started, I think. I used to tell my
husband there were ghosts there, just like a little child. He said, "Oh, that's
in your imagination. There's nothing in the attic that can hurt you." So he
even went up in the attic to show me that there was nothing to hurt me. I
don't know. I guess I got scared when I was little. In a convent these girls—
that's where I was raised—used to go around the dorms and scare us at
night. They'd say, "there's a redfaced man on the loose and he would get us,"
and oh God, we used to be scared half out of our wits.

Such intrinsic remedies may follow a presumption, later proved erroneous, that "she will snap out of it," or "I thought it would go away."

With the failure of intrinsic remedies to stop the advance of trouble
another attempted remedy was to change the environment. Since so
many of the trouble theories of these women and their husbands pivoted
around a notion of the need for rest, relaxation, or a change of scene,
vacations, the husband's changing or leaving his job (as in the case of
Louise Oren's earlier breakdown), or changing the wife's environment
were tried. The researchers reported: "One week before going to the
county hospital (prior to admission to Napa) Mrs. Arlen moved into her
mother's house. . . . After one week at her mother's house, she went to
the hospital. She told only her mother she was going, and she went there
herself in a taxi."

For some of the Bay Area families, psychiatric hospitalization represented the first involvement of professional outsiders in the remedial

cycle. For others, it occurred following less drastic forms of medical and psychiatric intervention. Three of the women had not seen a psychiatrist or psychologist prior to admission to Napa. Ten saw a psychiatrist one or more times during the preadmission crisis phase, while four had received treatment over a longer period: between eight and sixty-six sessions. If medical help was not sought prior to hospitalization, it was generally either because the husbands had not noticed anything was wrong, or because the families could not afford it.

The medical phase of the remedial cycle commonly began with a visit to the family doctor, who either attempted some treatment or referred the patient to a psychiatrist. Some patients received general-practitioner medical treatment and no outpatient psychiatric treatment, while others received both general and psychiatric care:

Joyce Noon: I then asked her how long she had been sick before she went into the hospital, and she said it was about two months. I asked her what she did about it, and she said "Nothing—I didn't know what to do about it." I then asked her if she saw a doctor, and she said, "Went to see my family doctor, he gave me some shots that didn't seem to work fast enough." She went on that instead of getting better, she was getting worse. I asked her what the doctor told her was wrong, and she said she didn't know either. I then asked her how she knew she was sick, or how she was sick. She said "Sick in the head—sick all over." I asked her to tell me more about this. "My whole body—head too—so it started to get where I couldn't sleep at night, but didn't know what it was, but knew it was something, so after two months of it decided to go to the hospital."

The search for expert remedial intervention was not always successful: in the family and social structure of the fifties, medical treatment of deviance was not so far advanced as readily to precipitate poorly functioning housewives into the sick role (Conrad and Schneider 1980). Troubles were liable to be ignored or minimized by doctors and husbands alike. Thus, two of the women reported that doctors initially refused to regard their troubles as psychiatric in nature. For example, Joyce Noon said that "The doctor she went to when she was troubled told her, 'You're young and healthy and you only have one boy—go home and take care of him.'"

Eventually, however, all these women's troubles came to be seen as psychiatric. And, as Erving Goffman notes, the addition of third parties into the marital dyad in the search for trouble remedies may be experienced by the troubled partner as a form of betrayal, both because it is seen as an "alienative coalition" and because it contributes to the definition of the patient as someone who cannot take care of her own problems (1961). As John Clausen and Marian Yarrow point out, "There is an ethic of being able to handle one's own problems by oneself, which applies not only to psychiatric problems" (1955, 26). And, as Derek Phillips notes, "the utilization of certain help-sources involves not only a reward (positive mental health) but also a cost (rejection by others, and consequently, a negative self-image)" (1963, 972). Furthermore, in the fifties family the wife's dependence on her husband implicated him in her troubles; seeking outside help implied that he could not care for or control his own family. Thus the search for outside help in remedying troubles in these families was limited by marital denial, cost factors, and the cultural emphasis on individual and familial self-help. But in the end, in each case, psychiatric hospitalization was accepted as a last-resort remedy for these women's troubles.

THE LAST STRAW

Some research attention has been paid to the "last straw" (Smith et al. 1963) that precipitates hospitalization as the "last resort" (Emerson 1981) of the remedial cycle. There are two kinds of crises that typically precede hospitalization: those which convince family members to commit their intimates or persuade them to sign themselves in, and those which convince the troubled to seek admission voluntarily. Kathleen Smith, Muriel Pumphrey, and Julian Hall studied last straws of the first kind and concluded:

[In the] 100 final decisive incidents . . . behavior was seen as: a) actually or potentially harmful . . . b) socially unacceptable . . . c) indicating mental illness and requiring treatment. . . . The 'last straws' were quite varied and bore no statistically significant relationship to age, sex, race, marital status, religion [etc.]. . . . Nine types of events had been tolerated frequently without a request for hospitalization: suicidal threats, threats of harm to family members, destructiveness, shouting, obscene words, irrational talk, inexplicable behavior, wandering, and refusing to come out of a room. Suicidal attempts and actual harm to others were not tolerated. (1963, 229)

For the Bay Area husbands, as for the family members in the Smith sample, the most common event immediately precipitating hospitalization was bizarre, inexplicable, or dangerous behavior. A majority of the Bay Area husbands reported that their wives were behaving bizarrely or dangerously, or were hallucinating or delusional, immediately prior to hospitalization (Warren 1983). For the Bay Area wives, the most common last straw was a crisis or cumulation of strange feelings, troubling thoughts, or weird behavior.

Dangerous behavior generally involved things emblematic of the role of housewife: destroying the household (selling furniture, setting the house on fire) or harming the children. Mr. Karr's wife "got loud, swearing, also expressing fears of harming the new baby by squeezing its ribs too hard. Disturbed the children by preaching religion." Mr. Oren found his wife breathing into the mouth of their three year-old-daughter and became quite concerned about her condition. Others made similar reports:

Mr. Thorne: "Happened while I was at work . . . the morning she choked [daughter] I had breakfast with her . . . she wasn't wrought up or anything like that. Then I got this call, my daughter was at a neighbor's house—she was strangling her" . . . [earlier she] "drank her coffee which had poison in it—strychnine—and I drank mine—she said I'm going to mail a letter, she gets in the car and drives off (to the mental hospital, as it later turns out). I didn't think anything was wrong . . . the neighbors would just kind of keep it to themselves, and I guess they figured I knew what was going on—I didn't."

A variety of bizarre as well as dangerous actions were reported by the husbands. Mrs. Oren was "knocking on doors" of neighbors with no apparent reason. And Mr. Quinn said, "I came home on the 14th of July and found she had defaced one of my daughter's dolls. I asked her why, and she said it was nobody's business. . . . She had broken a vase . . . she had taken this whistle and blown that thing for five minutes outside."

In the separate-worlds marriages, the last straw seemed to function as a means of communicating the woman's distress. The expression of extreme psychiatric symptoms and the search for medical intervention can be seen as ways of obtaining needed attention that had previously been denied. It is not clear just how consciously some of these women attempted to communicate their distress by becoming mental patients, but their actions certainly had that effect:

Mr Baker would accuse his wife of being an "unfit wife" and of being "crazy." She would admit this, saying, "I know I'm crazy, why don't you help me?" . . . Through insisting that if she went home she might "do something" to her children or herself. Mrs Baker convinced a physician that he should take immediate action in hospitalizing her. On the day of her admission, she told the interviewer: "my husband has to know about this or it isn't going to help me much."

Mrs Rand suffered from a variety of somatic complaints and a sense of impending personal disorganization for about two years prior to hospitalization. When she attempted to communicate her distress to her husband, he minimized her concerns, emphasized the demands placed on him by his work, and urged her not to bother him. . . . A few weeks later, Mrs Rand . . . arose at dawn, wrote her husband a brief note, and drove to church. She entered the minister's office, said, "God help me," and dissolved into tears. Once again, when the minister wanted to call her husband, she urged not disturbing him. Within an hour a worried and concerned husband was at her side and arrangements were underway to hospitalize her. During and after hospitalization Mrs Rand commented that her husband no longer ignored her, and seemed concerned with her feelings. (Messinger n.d., 18, 50)

Some of these women's dramatic communications were highly symbolic, such as Kate White's placing her wedding ring on the altar of her church (Sampson et al. 1964, 54).

The wives experienced frightening feelings and desires to harm themselves or others, delusions, or hallucinations as the last straws that led them to seek hospitalization. A few reported that they engaged in harmful or destructive behavior, including setting fire to the house, trying to choke a child, giving a tranquilizer pill to a child, and attempting suicide. For Cora Thorne, one violent act led to a feeling of despair that precipitated another:

I asked her if she had experienced any kind of emotional upset or difficulty before this. "I don't know—nothing like this—just too many things thrown at me at one time—I just lost self-control—I panicked." (In what way did you panic?) "I talked too much . . . I said too many things to too many people—I tried to get too much advice—but instead I lost everything—friends, relatives, everything." I asked her what had happened that led her to going to the county hospital. "I tried to choke my little girl—but I panicked in the end—and stopped." (Why did you try to choke her?) "Because I thought that when she and the little boy went to school, they would be told that their momma was in the hospital because she tried to kill herself."

Cora was among a number of the women who felt uncontrollable despair and anger.

Shirley Arlen: Questioning elicited that it was Mrs. Arlen's decision to go to [the mental hospital]. "I did not want to die, and I felt I would kill myself."

Rose Price: "I realized I'd better be getting help" because "I knew I was going to do something bad . . . I went down and I told (Welfare) I don't want them coming to my door for any reason and that if they did I would kill them. . . . When I hurt myself by banging my arms against the wall I'm hurting them. . . . Was pregnant at time of admission to [hospital] and miscarried soon after."

Other women reported that the strangeness of their feelings, their "sickness" itself, was enough to make them request admission. In describing an earlier crisis that did not end in hospitalization, Ann Rand said that she was "missing the ironing board," then found it "standing right up in the kitchen. It frightened me. I felt I had wandered around in a daze" (Sampson et al. 1964, 78). She had wanted to go to the mental hospital, but her husband talked her out of it.

But husbands were not always so dilatory. In some cases, the husbands' involvement in their wives' search for psychiatric help came about not because of a behavioral last straw but because of their wives' communication of extreme distress:

Nelson White: He said his wife had entered . . . hospital after becoming upset sometime during the Easter season. She had been going to a psychiatrist for somewhat over a year. She began to see a psychiatrist when she felt that something had snapped inside her head. She felt that this had been caused by herself. . . . Mr. White indicated that he had gotten into treatment with a psychiatrist too.

Other wives experienced a crisis in their feelings and sought assistance from their husbands:

Eve Low: She traced it back to January 1958, but then said, "no, it really started on December 15, 1957," and launched into a story about some incident with her cousin on that day. Then, or shortly afterward, she woke up at night feeling very sick and told her husband to get a doctor, "that I was going crazy. That my feet burned. I took a hot bath."

Although marital troubles were seen by many of the women as contributing to their emotional distress, none were as clear about the causal
relationship as Peggy Sand. For Peggy, Napa represented one in a long
series of places to which she would sporadically run from Floyd. Her
account of the circumstances of her hospitalization makes an interesting
contrast with her admission notes:

(Peggy Sand, admitted May 8, 1958, last child born May 8, 1952; first
interview 5.11.58) Dr. H notes: "grimly smiling and sublimely blinking
married woman who has just had too much in the home situation in the past
few months. Depressed and confused but not depersonalized, apparently.
Oriented, coherent, tense inside. BP normal. No recent infections. Impression: reactive depression."

When I asked her why she came into Napa, she said that she didn't know
where else to turn . . . I asked her again what prompted her to come in . . .
and she said, "well, I would say, marital problems." She said that her
husband was very domineering and critical, and it got to the point where
she couldn't take any more. She felt that if she stayed she thought that she
might have bashed her husband's head in. [Later] she said that she came here
to the hospital to either learn to live with him, or else to learn how to stand
up to him. She said that she hoped she could be a better mother when she
left the hospital. I asked her if anything special had been happening recently
to her. She said there was nothing special, although things had not been
good for quite some time. She described one incident, about a month ago,
when her husband had been drinking this particular night and he came in
and "he hurt me." She "was going to run away." But she was "too tired . . .
didn't have the energy to get in the car and leave."

In a subsequent interview, she described how she literally escaped to
Napa from her husband:

[Some salesmen were selling frozen meat, and instead of telling them to go
away she told them to come back when her husband was home]. Then the
salesmen came back to talk to her husband about frozen food. Her husband

told the salesmen they were not interested in it. Then her husband came back and "turned to me. . . . He said, 'if someone came to the door and said he was interested in pussy, you'd give it to him.'" She said, "that did it. . . . He's told me worse things before, but that was the last straw." She said she took the car and went to Napa.

As these comments indicate, the Sands were among the several couples whose lives were characterized by marital violence. But violence of husband against wife was not interpreted by either spouse as symptomatic of mental illness. Indeed, the husbands were inclined to view physical assaults on their wives as a form of legitimate punishment: Mel Noon and two other husbands beat up or tried to strangle their wives for suspected involvements with other men (in each case by the man's own account). But violence on the part of wives was construed as abnormal, indeed as bizarre and dangerous, and thus as a symptom of mental illness. Mr. Yale said that one factor precipitating his wife's hospitalization was that she would hit him when they argued. Similarly, Mr. Vick described the last straw prior to his wife's hospitalization, when "she threw a steam iron at him—missed him, and barely missed his mother. Rita then called the police to take her to the psychiatric hospital. 'She said that she was crazy or something.'"

It is clear from these accounts that the last straw prior to hospitalization reflected woman's place in the fifties family in ways that were quantitatively but not qualitatively different from her routine violations of the housewife role. Even the bizarre and dangerous acts she engaged in reflected the madwife's distress as a traditional woman. She physically attacked her husband or children or repudiated them with dramatic symbolism. She burned her house, broke her dishes, or smashed her children's dolls. And then she went to the mental hospital.

How Did It Happen?

In the first few interviews, the day or week of first hospitalization, the Bay Area interviewers asked the respondents to account for the troubles that had brought the women to Napa. The husbands in particular gave answers that already bore the stamp of psychiatric interpretation, in their identification of both situational and deeper causes. Among the situational causes the respondents cited not only the troublesome aspects of the housewife role noted in the previous chapter, but also troubles related to the woman's place in her other social circles: the extended family, the neighborhood, and the network of social institutions that represented the larger society in the experience of these families. The roles in which troubles were experienced included those of daughter, mother, neighbor, wife, citizen, and family member.

The original researchers traced the deeper causes of hospitalization to the woman's relationship with her mother as it was echoed in her marital relationship. For example, the researchers analyzed June Mark, Donna Urey, and Irene James as having undergone "crises of identification" in which

marital life . . . reproduced a situation which corresponded to an earlier turning point in the wives' relations to their mothers. This repetition mobilized dissociated identifications with a characteristic content. This content included the mother as victim and as object of the child's anger. It also included the child as evilly responsible for the maternal loss and as a confused, helpless and deprived victim. This constellation of parent–child identification was warded off until marital life revived it and undermined the previous defensive position. (Sampson et al. 1964, 59)

During the course of hospitalization, a number of the women learned to apply this psychological theory of causes rooted in their original families, blaming their mothers (and sometimes fathers) for their emotional troubles (see chapter 7). But in the first few interviews the focus was not on parents. Rather—and especially among those women with paranoid delusions—it was on neighbors.

Only a minority of the Bay Area women lived with or close to their extended families; all lived in close proximity to neighbors. The meaning of neighbors in these women's everyday lives was in many ways more salient than the meaning of parents, at least overtly. Neighbors might be friends or acquaintances. Neighbors functioned as indicators of the family's status in the community and—insofar as the neighborhood was a reflection of the status system in the society as a whole—of their place in the world. Neighbors could represent a friendly refuge from marital incompatibility or a hostile and rebuffing environment for couples sensitive about their poverty or class origins and about the place of their children in the world. Troubles with neighbors reflected these themes, from Mary Yale's and Kate White's accusations of "homosexuality" against a female neighbor to the paranoia expressed by Louise Oren and Eve Low. In Mr. Oren's explanation of his wife's breakdown:

He talked about things that had happened in the tract where they lived, the fact that the house "depressed" her. . . . He said that once in the past his wife had seen their little girl get pushed around by a neighbor kid. . . . Finally, she spoke to the other kid's mother about it, who said, "go tell a cop." . . . He went on to say that sometimes at parties people would have a few drinks and say things to her that would hurt her.

Only one respondent traced her troubles to persons within the institutional structure of society rather than those within her intimate social circles:

Rita Vick: "I feel that it is Welfare that has really driven me to this place. Maybe I'm wrong, but it's my impression that Welfare is to help you, not to knock you down. They made me feel I'm no good to my children or to myself. That's why I'm here today. It isn't on account of my childhood. Some people say it's my childhood. Maybe it has something to do with it—I don't know."

Despite their place in the fifties family, none attributed their difficulties to structural factors beyond their control or that of their immediate social circles. This fact is of course not surprising in a culture that represents troubles as rooted in individual flaws and in private struggles. The medical model of mental illness encourages those labeled as mad to search for deeper as well as situational causes of their difficulties and to search for them within their individual experiences. Over time, the Bay Area women learned to trace their troubles farther back than to their neighbors, marriages, or children to their early childhood (this theme will be developed in chapter 7, but for now we are concerned with earlier accounts). The husbands seemed to learn the lessons of psychiatric biography more readily; even in the first few interviews they proffered psychiatric explanations for their wives' troubles, generally psychological but sometimes somatic. Mr. Quinn, for example, proposed a hereditary theory in this first interview:

I then asked, "How did it all start?" He sat back in his chair, looked thoughtful, and then said "Well (pause), I personally believe it started in her birthright somewhere along the line. I don't believe this is a manipulative thing. I believe it's a breakdown of the mind. It's a hard thing to define but I certainly think it must be tissue damage to start with or something wrong."

Whether the deeper cause was psychological or somatic in the husbands' view, they saw it as giving rise to enduring personality flaws in the woman, which created trouble for her in her marriage and other social relationships. The application of the medical model taught these men and women that it was not the social context that was defective but the deviating individual. Thus the protest and the movements toward independence of such women as Mary Yale and Kate White were interpreted as an aberrantly "masculine" personality caused by early childhood experiences (see Sampson et al. 1964). And the cumulation of experience only inventoried personal flaws. Not only the men but also the women saw their biographies in these ways:

Rita Vick: (Where did it start?) "You mean when I got sick, like, the tantrums like?" (Yes). "Well, when I was a child, my parents were awfully strict. I was not allowed to do anything. I was very quiet and would never talk back to anyone. I got married in 1948. I was divorced in 1950. I was twenty years old when I got married. After my divorce, I started being belligerent with people. I still am. I still have the fear—I feel that I'm being cut, and I have to fight back. . . . By being belligerent, I felt I was strong. Then three years ago I lost custody of my oldest child. . . . That hit me hard. It did something to me. . . . All I remember is that when I came to I was in a straitjacket, in . . . hospital."

From the husband's perspective, the wife's personality flaws were the beginning of a lifelong deterioration. They saw their wives' troubles as having proceeded through a series of cumulative stages, with different causative elements entering in and making her progressively worse. Mr. Quinn, in the same interview in which he referred to his wife's mental illness as her "birthright," continued:

(When did you first notice that something was wrong?) "It's hard to say (pause). I think I first noticed things were wrong when our second child was born . . . she's an alcoholic you know." . . . (Did she drink from the time you married her?) "No, it wasn't right from the beginning. Oh she drank socially. I guess a person is born with a weakness for that sort of thing and it accelerated. The whole thing seems to hinge with me on after the baby was born. After that time things really got rough. I was home when the boy was born but I left and didn't see him again until he was a year old. I was in the Navy four years."

Mr. Quinn seemed to be aware of the shifting nature of biographical interpretations. He said, "There again I have had so many definitions of her . . . but then again I was a lot younger and a lot less wiser than I am now. And I think, to reflect back 11 years is a hard task."

During the course of hospitalization, the women learned to create coherent biographies based on psychiatric principles and to locate their troubles in a natural history. But most did not do so during the first few weeks of hospitalization; instead, their accounts of "what happened" were highly situational, shifting, and sometimes incoherent. In the first three interviews, for example, Louise Oren referred to a variety of factors from physical ailments to moving as responsible for her troubles:

(3/13/58—voluntary admissions accompanied by husband): She is preoccupied with somatic symptoms and told me she has 'female trouble.' She repeatedly told me "it's hard to talk. I wish I could talk. My throat is so dry." She also complained of severe pains in her chest. When I asked how she happened to decide to come to Napa, she blocked severely and appeared deeply troubled.

(3/17/58): "Dr. H. wanted me to go there for research." . . . The trouble started "when we first moved in" (to a new house), and then she reversed herself saying, "not when I first moved in." She stopped to think a bit, and then asked, "you are not a newspaper reporter are you?" I told her I was not, and also reassured her about the confidentiality of what she was saying. Mrs. Oren then continued in a somewhat disconnected fashion. She talked about when they had first moved in, they had nice neighbors, and there were phrases about someone asking questions about parties, and getting a telephone call from the sheriff, who wanted to know the names of some people. "Anyway, I got a check—it was forged—had my name on it" . . . I asked her a question about anybody wanting to harm her. She said, "to harm—yeah, the children."

(3/24/58): "I signed myself in. Sometimes I felt I talk too much—it's hard to talk about such things." She went on to say that she tries to forget, and that she also has "mental blocks."

(4/24/58): I asked Mrs. Oren why she had gone to Napa. She said, "hadn't slept the night before, Dr. M. saw me—got a shot—couldn't rest—got to Napa, place to rest for a while—now all rested up."

The natural history of an episode of trouble also varies with the tellers, in this case husbands and wives. Mr. Oren gave a rather different account of Louise's troubles than did his wife:

"I didn't notice too much after that (a prior "breakdown" four or five years ago) but the neighbors did." Mr. Oren then described how his wife would call up the neighbors next door and speak in a rather high pitched voice. . . . "Then—check business—sheriff came to home about check . . . neighbors." The sheriff then told Mrs. Oren that this boy, who is either the son of the neighbor or the neighbor himself, and was twenty-one years old . . . was a homosexual. This disturbed the wife very much as their children had often gone over to this particular neighbor's house to play. The sheriff also said he believed there was a house of "ill fame" operating across the street.

The women learned over time to look beyond personality flaws for the deeper causes of their troubles. Even at this early stage of theorizing, the women patterned their difficulties into sequences, which were then linked to historical precedents:

Wanda Karr: I asked her whether the patient had ever had similar experiences in the past to that which she now was having. "I had to quit school about five times for my nerves. Wish mama'd put me in the hospital then. I was a lot calmer then . . . I was a wreck, I would just get so upset." (Cry?) "Day and night. I couldn't eat; I'd throw up . . . Mama just made me quit school. She said I'd make myself crazy studying and all. . . . Dr. P. could tell I got upset while carrying the baby."

In tracing historical precedents for their current sequence of trouble, both Wanda Karr and Peggy Sand reported dependency and control relations in their family of origin similar to those they later experienced with their husbands. Both linked the escalation of troubles to these circumstances:

Peggy Sand: Said that she married at 17 and implied this might have been a desire to get away from her mother, who she described as being "bossy," and said her husband was the same way.

Wanda Karr: (Was the upset the same before?) "It was worse before I was married. When I got married things changed. My folks wouldn't let me go anyplace. Boys . . . they wouldn't let me go out at all. . . . After marriage it was different, my folks didn't trust me before . . . Richard's the only boy I ever went with."

The process of theorizing trouble and the biographical work that accompanied it continued throughout the patient and ex-patient stages of the moral career. Although it had a "natural history" aspect it was also highly situational; facets of life or self seen as trouble-causing in an unhappy moment may not be viewed in the same spirit during a happy one. Furthermore, as some of the respondents recognized, the context of theorizing can transform the past more than once. According to Mr. Rand, "While she [wife] was here in the hospital she would think what an unhappy childhood she had, but when she was out of the hospital she would think of how happy a childhood it was."

Over time, as we will see in chapter 6, some of the husbands learned to place the blame for their wives' hospitalization on the marital relationship or on their own behavior. In particular, they came to understand the strain of the housewife role. But in the first few interviews only Mr. White saw his own behavior as precipitating the crisis of hospitalization and his own personality flaws as creating their marital difficulties. In the first interview, on 12 November 1957, he blamed his wife's hospitalization on his being "fat, lazy and unconcerned," and on his job changes. In the next interview he cited his own peculiar psychology as contributing to the couple's current predicament:

Mr White indicated that he had thought of something unusual the other night. It had to do with his attraction to unusual gals. . . . In college he went with one whom he thought was probably emotionally disturbed . . . "they all seemed different. I didn't think about this before." He then talked about something he knew troubled his wife a great deal. To settle down was always a problem for him. They moved about a great deal and he could never commit himself to one thing or another.

Although Kate White's hospitalization may have been Nelson White's "fault," it nevertheless still reflected deviations from the gender-role structure of the fifties family: the "gals" he was attracted to were "unusual" in their independence and thus probably "disturbed," while he was "unusual" in his lack of commitment to adult breadwinner roles, and thus equally open to suspicion.

Gender roles in the fifties, and in particular the housewife role, provide the biographical and historical key to understanding the social situation of the madwife. The strain of the female role precipitated emotional distress; in turn, trouble was defined as emotional by virtue of inadequate performance of that role. Hospitalization occurred in the wake of failed remedial action. And with the inception of a new, psychiatric (auto)biography, the critique of social structure implicit in these women's distress was, for the time being, effectively silenced.

The Mental Patient

CHAPTER 4

In the Mental Hospital

In the mental hospital, the housewife becomes a mental patient. But the adoption of the sick role does not mean that other roles are erased; instead, both prior and current experiences shape patients' interpretations of what is happening to them. On entering Napa, the Bay Area patient took with her the structure of her marital relationship, with its typical patterns of dominance and submission, power and dependence. At the same time, she encountered a world with its own structure, its own patterns of authority and subordination. Housework, work outside the home, money, and sex were themes elaborated in the mental hospital, as well as out of it.

First, in view of the strain and boredom of the housewife role and the isolation of these women, the mental hospital provided something of a refuge or moratorium for the incarcerated housewife (see also Sampson et al. 1964), an ironic countrast to the literature on the coercive asylum (Goffman 1961; Perruci 1974; but see Braginsky et al. 1969). But at the same time the hospital also provided a context in which prior roles could be lived out, for example by doing housework on the ward or by nurturing other patients.

The hospital experience both shored up and undermined the expectations of women who came from the traditional fifties family. Women who wanted to work outside the home in a career found themselves able to do such work at Napa, in the hospital beauty shop, radio station, or newspaper room. But at the same time, hospitalization was structured, medically and legally, to supplement marital control with psychiatric. The discharge conference, by which the Bay Area women were restored

95

to their place in the family, exemplified this dual control. And, in a different way, so did the plight of the madwife facing separation from her husband and (sometimes) children. Thus, hospitalization was experienced through the lens of the historical self and its current roles and relationships in the traditional family. Furthermore, there were the practicalities of these roles and relationships to contend with: despite the Bay Area women's hospitalization, there was still housework to be done and child care to be arranged. Although the Bay Area husbands generally transferred these functions to the female kin network, the wives were left with a sense of guilt at having betrayed their husbands and (particularly) children by mental hospitalization, and they felt a pervasive anxiety concerning the care given by substitutes.

It is not surprising that the sum of these experiences in the mental hospital gave rise to some ambivalence about leaving. Mental hospitalization provided the madwife with things that she did not get in everyday life and that she wanted very badly; but at the same time it took away the anchors to that everyday life on which her very identity depended.

The Mental Hospital as a Refuge

The vast literature on the sick role is focused around the idea of refuge; that to be labeled physically or mentally ill provides the individual with a way to escape his or her ordinary role demands. In the case of the fifties housewife, it appears that the sick role itself did not necessarily provide a refuge; rather, it was the mental hospital that did so. The meaning of the sick role proved to be somewhat ambiguous, both in and out of the mental hospital.

As Harold Sampson, Sheldon Messinger, and Robert Towne note in their book on the Bay Area women, the hospital experience functions as "time out" from the constant demands and pressures of the housewife's everyday life (1964). A number of the women expressed their sense of relief at the "rest" provided by their stay at Napa. They experienced a moratorium on the strains and complexities of housewifery and the marital relationship. Joyce Noon expressed this idea on various occasions:

She indicated that she might like to go home every now and then and see the family, and then go back to the hospital to "rest." This would be better for her son than divorce.

"You start resting and eating and completely different surroundings, it does you a world of good. You forget. . . . At home. . . . You're just stuck with it."

"I like it here [Napa]—I'm getting used to it—I go out (on home visits) whenever I think I can and then when it's too much for me I come back in. . . . I'm not even trying to get of out being married or anything. I gave up—but he should . . . know that. He thinks that he has to keep on, you know, as if I didn't give up."

The lack of communication with their husbands experienced by these women and their isolation from the company of their families or others during the day was partially compensated for at Napa. The theme of the hospital as lessening isolation and increasing both communication and the sense of communicative competence was expressed by several patients, including Mary Yale: "At one point she said she had learned a lot here, the patients understand, and she sees in the patients the things that are true of herself also, which is very helpful. Also she likes to hear them talk. 'It's very educational.' She never hears people talk like this outside. 'It's very stimulating.'"

Schizophrenia, and madness in general, is archaically named alienation, and the psychiatrists who seek to alleviate these conditions, alienists. In the mental hospital, these women had some opportunity to become less alienated from their sense of self, their egos, because they were temporarily removed from the isolated dependence that was at the root of alienation. As the comments above indicate, at Napa the women not only "had a rest," they also learned that they were not alone, that others shared the same problems and pleasures. Peggy Sand commented, after one of her several hospitalization episodes:

"He says I'm sick, sick, sick, can't think straight, don't know what I'm doing, I've been sick all these years and never stopped to analyze it." At which she laughed. Then she suddenly buried her head in her hands, and seemed to be sobbing, although I couldn't tell for sure. After about half-a-minute or so, she looked up again and was fairly composed. She then said that "in a way perhaps I have been." I asked her about this. "Oh, insecurity, not having anyone to turn to, talk to, not having anyone to build my ego up, instead of knocking it down, dragging it down, not to know who to turn to, where to go."

In place of the housewife role, the schizophrenic woman temporarily occupied the sick role. In the fifties family assuming this role did not give her much relief from household responsibilities until she was actually removed from the household as a mental patient. Being emotionally disturbed was not, in the fifties, an excuse for not doing the ironing or making dinner. The instruction to "snap out of it" was part of the prepatient experience of most of the Bay Area women.

Once hospitalized, the role demands of the traditional household ceased—or at least took a different form. But the sick role did not release the patients from taking responsibility for their own welfare. At Napa in the fifties, the practice of medicine involved a stress on the self, as against doctors, as the source of help. For the Bay Area patients, the "affliction and therapy" model coexisted uneasily with the "individual effort" model; there was considerable puzzlement over the fact that they were repeatedly told that the doctors were not there to cure them. As Joyce Noon complained, "The nurse . . . said [the doctor] isn't going to cure you. . . . You have to cure yourself, something like that." Not surprisingly, the patients wondered why they were in a mental hospital if they had to cure themselves.

The Bay Area husbands seemed to concur in the hospital's injunctions to wifely self-reliance. The husbands were also told that it was up to the wives rather than the doctors to "get better." Further, self-will as a means to change behavior and mood is a popular theme in our culture (even more in the eighties than the fifties) and had been among the remedial repertoire of the respondents prior to the Napa episode. Thus Mr. James said:

he thinks if she would try harder she would improve a lot more. It was clear that he blames her to some extent for not making sufficient effort . . . he remarked with a slight humorous laugh that he hates to call it laziness but. He paused a moment and then said he probably should call it mental laziness. He went on to say, however, that really she has always been this way.

The wives were uncertain about where they stood. Since many of them suffered from troubling feelings and thoughts, they were inclined—particularly at their most troubled moments—to claim the sick role. But on the other hand they were not unaffected by the cultural, medical, and marital calls to self-reliance. So they wavered:

Ruth Quinn: "He doesn't understand mental illness . . . he doesn't understand I'm not responsible. He just doesn't understand." But earlier she had said, "I've stopped my crying and that's good. I have a great feeling of individuality and having to do it on your own. I think that is the way to get out of here [Napa] rather than the jobs you do or the time you are here."

As this comment indicates, the Bay Area women were also aware of the potential of displays of self-reliance for controlling the kind of impression they made in the hospital. Whether they felt self-reliant or not, they attempted to display signs of self-control (mainly by not crying), independence, and "trying" in their everyday life on the ward. That way, they reasoned, lay freedom.

Displays of self-as-resource were also sometimes directed at the husbands, and at other times even at themselves. Ruth Quinn reported that her sister had advised her, "if you are very cautious about not crying on the phone, he will be much more apt to let you see the children." In the ex-patient phase, while separated from her husband, Ruth had problems getting up in the morning. She said then, "I decided that the best thing I can do is to just use self-discipline to get myself out. And eventually it will become a pattern just like it was up there [Napa]. And eventually I'll feel better and learn self-respect and self-reliance." Self-discipline and self-control became the ways in which getting better was made possible, or at least discharge was obtained.

The respite from housework, the contact with other women, and the focus on the self—its power and its unique history—were highly contradictory features of mental hospital life in the fifties. The overt messages of hospitalization, which involved the restoration of women to the housewife role (and, presumably, of men to that of breadwinner) were consistently undermined by the more covert ones. The same might be said of those social arrangements by which Napa State Hospital arranged the everyday lives of patients in the fifties: their work and leisure activities.

WORK AND LEISURE

The round of daily events at Napa had its own institutional logic, but it also had implications for the historical self of the mental patient: for her prior and future roles and relationships within the family. The institutional logic of hospital work has been documented in ethnographies. Although the practice is clothed in the therapeutic rhetoric of "occupational therapy," patients labor in the mental hospital in order to keep the institution running. The logic of hospital leisure is similarly framed: the numerous leisure activities provoked at Napa in the fifties enabled staff to keep patients busy, and thus promoted preventive ward control. But the meaning of work and leisure in the mental hospital was, for the Bay Area patients, embedded in the context of their place as women in the fifties family; neither therapy nor ward control could adequately summarize what Napa's routines meant to them.

Like most institutions, Napa depended on patient labor for much of its day-to-day "household" operation. And like the staff of most institutions—in the eighties as in the fifties—the Napa staff justified using patient housework labor as a therapeutic device that could teach or reinforce attention to outside stimuli over the internal stimuli of schizophrenia. Though phrased in therapeutic terms, the function of ward work was to ease everyday chores for the staff. Patients who were cooperative were rewarded by discharge. One interviewer commented:

I discovered that both the Dr.'s ideas and the techs as to how a patient can get off S-6 [ward] relates [sic] to the patient's willingness to do 'work.' The patient has to first show interest in work on the ward before she is even recommended . . . for off-ward work. As the tech put it, "if the patient can't do a little work on the ward one can't predict that she will do any better on off-ward work or at home." And 'getting home' is not only contingent on an 'appropriate receiver' but evidence is needed that the patient is willing and able to work in order to pass at conference. Dr. C said that work experience and a P-card [card indicating the patient has grounds and other privileges] "look awfully good" at the conference. If a patient doesn't have these—it is questionable that she will get out.

The response of the patients to the housework demands made on them reflected their sense of place. Patients refused or resented housework demands either if they felt too ill to do such work or if they had learned to resent it. Their in-hospital role performance tended to mirror their prehospital behavior, whether lying in bed all day neglecting chores or doing chores fretfully. In some cases, women who performed housework adequately and without resentment in their homes became angry at Napa because of the work's connotation of indentured labor; however, this response was rare in this mainly lower-class sample:

Rita Vick: She said she had to do some ward work. . . . She had worked all morning on beds and had to tie bundles in the afternoon. . . . She said the nurses "pick on you" to work. Only about three or four on the ward do any. . . . (What is your feeling about ward work?) "I don't want to work, I'm tired of it. I have to fix shock beds all morning and tie bundles in the afternoon."

Other women—or the same women in different moods—welcomed the ward work. It provided both a relief from boredom and inactivity and a way of reminding the women that they were not useless, that their role loss in the hospital could be mitigated. Among these women were a number whose housework on the wards generally exceeded the demands placed on them by staff. They were not working only to please staff or to show that they were better; their motivation also expressed the preservation of their historical selves in this new setting. This response to ward work was often expressed as "keeping busy," as in a conversation with Rita Vick. Asked what had happened to her request for dining-room work, "She said it took a long time to work that out. But a patient on the ward had told her that she was in the hospital eleven years before working in the dining room—'I'd rather work at home.' She went on to say that 'work gives you glory—it makes you feel better.'"

For the wives who did housework in the hospital—who washed floors, made beds, cooked, or did the laundry—ward life represented in part an echo of, or a continuity with, their housewife selves. But for a number of the women, "outside" work in the hospital represented an alternative to the housewife roles they had become disenchanted with on the outside. Several of the women worked in the Napa hairdressing facility or as secretaries in the wards or offices. This type of "pink collar" work represented for some of the women either the potential that housewifery had never allowed them to develop, or half-buried aspects of their prehospital selves, or both. As Mary Yale said of her work as secretary on the OT ward, "it's good for me." She said that when people feel she does a good job, she enjoys a sense of validation; and it helps her keep busy and pass the time.

The highest positions in this hospital work hierarchy were reporting and writing for the *Imola News*, the hospital newspaper, or broadcasting for the hospital radio station. Kate White and Donna Urey, who eventually worked in these positions, had both been interested in finding work outside the home in their pre-Napa days but had husbands who did not "allow" them to work. Both women found an opportunity at Napa for the expression of talents and interests that they perceived as otherwise buried in their housewife roles. Kate White commented of her job at the *News* that "She was enjoying her work at the Imola News and it made her feel good to be back 'in harness' so to speak. I asked if she had thought of working again. She had and would very much like to work, but realized that it was very difficult being a photographer and a mother at the same time." The experience reminded Kate White of what her life had been like before marriage—to the detriment, in her view, of her current housewife role.

While these nonhousewife Napa working experiences were sometimes disturbing to the Bay Area women—in the sense of further disturbing any contentment with housewifery and the status quo—there were other Napa experiences that disturbed their spouses. Certain features of everyday life at Napa were symbolic of patients not as housewives (or in the case of male patients, wage earners) but as predomestic, sexual, desirable, partying, leisure-oriented and essentially youthful selves. As I noted in chapter 1, the state mental hospitals of the fifties were in some ways small self-contained societies. In addition to the work and therapeutic activities open to patients, there were numerous leisure pursuits available—far more numerous indeed than in their outside lives as housewives. In one interview with Donna Urey, for example, she mentioned the following: a hospital dance with a crowned Beauty Queen and court of twelve candidates (which included not only dancing and a band but acrobats, tap dancers, singers, and ballet dancers); indoor basketball, baseball, volleyball, badminton, and roller skating; movies; ward games including cards, crossword puzzles, and word games; outdoor trips to local swimming pools; and woodwork, plastics, and dressmaking. Many of these activities were pleasing to the patients in the straightforward senses of occupying time or testing competence, or in the symbolic sense of reorienting one's activities to the family. But others, most obviously the parties and dances, reminded these women of their prehousewife selves, which was a source of gratification to them but a threat to their husbands.

The Bay Area husbands complained bitterly about their wives' participation, without them, in cross-sex dancing and party activities at Napa. Donna Urey, having inventoried all the activities she could and did participate in, added that "when she's home she tells her husband about all the parties and dances she goes to here and he doesn't like it; he gets angry." Mel Noon complained that "his wife will 'doll up real nice' for the dances at Napa and ask him to bring her perfume, lipstick, etc." And Leo Vick expressed his sense of betrayal at the role reversal that Napa seemed to have precipitated in their domestic arrangements:

I sit alone every night . . . taking care of my kids and taking care of my house. And she's up there having a good time. . . . She's got two nice dresses up there—I mean party dresses—She's a married woman. What the hell do they run up there—a romance bureau or something? She's supposed to be over there for doctoring—instead she goes roller skating and to movies. She tells me whenever they have a dance.

As Goffman notes, flirtatious romance tends to flourish in the mental hospital (1961); at Napa, the term used was an "Imola romance." And certainly these husbands' objections and jealousies were justified from the perspective of maintaining the domestic status quo, since their wives' dissatisfaction with housewifery was underlined by these reminders of a more golden era (fantasized or otherwise) of the self. Some of the wives, however, behaving properly in role, limited their participation in Napa's cross-sex activities: the researchers reported that June Mark described how they had a Christmas party with five musicians and a table for cards and bingo, and dancing. "Although she 'feels funny' about dancing when her husband is not there she did 'a little.'"

The hospital experience became for these women a reminder of what they had been, or might have been, if they had not entered into their current marital and family status. Ward life and hospital activities were in a sense regressive to the predomestic past, producing a boarding-school or high-school atmosphere. At the same time, the self-analytic and past-oriented thrust of group or individual therapy could promote a critical comparison of one's past, present, and future prospects.

All the Bay Area women had a period in their past life, prior to this marriage, that was remembered or idealized as a golden age, free of troubles, when they were at their best. For most of the women this was in high school. Interestingly enough, three of them referred to their equality with boys in sports and other activities at this time as one of the features of this golden age; for Ann Rand, "When the girls were just as important as the boys." For two, the golden age was represented by earlier marriages to men who now seemed better or richer or at least less trouble than their current spouses. A few recalled earlier plans for a career. Joyce Noon, in describing her golden age, highlights both its hopeful quality and the contrast between her hopes and the realities of life for women in the fifties:

"When I was about 17 or 18 I had a lot of big ideas . . . I wanted to be a lab tech or something (laughs) . . . I don't know, great big things to do and everything, and I don't know it seems like most girls usually gravitate right into getting married anyway . . . it's the most natural thing to do . . . ideas of being an old maid. . . . It's a hard thing to do, be an old maid. . . . I thought I'd probably be a lab technician, get to go around and follow these ideas, you know . . . and I finally got married."

Marital and Psychiatric Control

The structure of mental hospitalization in the fifties had implications not only for the roles and selves of women patients, but also for their marital relationships. For women patients, the experience of mental hospitalization was essentially one in which their subordination was amplified by a coalition of marital and psychiatric authority. In the prepatient stage of the moral career, such a coalition had literally been formed; Goffman describes this process as the "betrayal funnel" by which one family member forces or persuades another into the mental hospital (1961). And in the mental hospital of the fifties, the reinforcement of marital with psychiatric control was continued through the staff's measurement of mental health by the restoration of the housewife role and the marital relationship. The women recognized their situation and resented it: Joyce Noon says, on being asked why she has been readmitted, "Every time you ask me that you have to ask him [husband] because I don't know what he's doing . . . [he] doesn't feel secure unless I'm under some authority . . . as long as I'm his wife he can do with me as he pleases. . . . I cannot fight him . . . he will not let me work and he put me under these authorities." Shirley Arlen complained:

"I just don't see how they could go ahead and stick me under his thumb like that—for that's what it amounts to." I asked her if this was something she thought they deliberately tried to do. "I don't know—I wouldn't like to say that—at the same time, that's what it all amounts to." I asked her if she feels now that she is pretty much under her husband's control. "Yeah." (More so than when you went into the hospital) "More so—yes." (In just what ways?) "Because whenever he takes a darn good notion—he can take me right back there—or call and have me picked me up—although he may not be able to keep me there." (Do you think he would do this?) "I wouldn't be surprised if he did." (What kind of circumstances might cause him to do that?) "I think the minute I went and filed for divorce, that's exactly what he'll do." (Just what are you going to do with the situation?) She stared ahead reflectively and then answered, "I'll probably just go on like I did before. What else is there to do? He doesn't want me to go to work—" (Why doesn't he?) "He says he doesn't want me to have to work—besides which I belong here with the kids."

The mental hospital of the fifties quite explicitly used the marital relationship and the housewife role as criteria for mental-health assessments and as part of the discharge decision. After "failing" discharge conferences a second time, Kate White, who had earlier told the interviewer she had finally learned "what to say," was successful in her attempts to be discharged once she declared that her marital relationship was improved and that hospitalization had helped her: "Dr. B. then asked 'Do you think your hospitalization has helped you any?' Mrs. White: 'It sure has.' 'How do you and your husband get along now?' 'Wonderful.' 'Better.' 'We sure do'" (indefinite leave, 4/1/59). Peggy

Sand's three discharge conferences exemplify the hospital's use of the marital relationship and role criteria in psychiatric decision making. The following are excerpts from each of these conferences:

(first discharge conference, 7/30/58)—*Dr. C:* "Why are you here?" *Peggy Sand:* "My husband signed a petition to have me committed." *Dr. C.:* "Does he think you are crazy?" *Peggy Sand:* "The hospital asked him before if he thought I was crazy and he said no. Then he said that the people at the hospital told me that I was sick enough to be committed." *Dr. C.:* "Do you get along with him now, or do you still fight?" *Peggy Sand:* "I can get along with him after a fashion . . . for the time being I'll go home to him. I've been placed in a position where I'm dependent upon him for everything I do." *Dr. R.:* "What do you mean 'go back home'?" *Peggy Sand:* "Oh, be a housewife, cook the meals, take care of the children." *Dr. D.:* "How do you picture your future?" *Peggy Sand:* "Very bleak" (she said this in a matter of fact way, but then her voice cracked and she appeared and sounded a little more depressed and almost on verge of tears). "But I'm tired of beating my head on a stone wall." *Dr. D.:* "You say everything depends on him—how?" *Peggy Sand:* (She said something to the effect that, in the first place, she was married to him, and now she is in here and he has so much say over things that happen to her. . . . Later, after Peggy Sand had left the room): After a brief pause, Dr. B. asked Dr. D. what she thought. She answered, "You mean, is she psychotic?—oh I don't think so." Dr. C. immediately chimed in "I don't think she is psychotic either." However Dr. McG. said, "I think she is schizophrenic." He added that she probably has had a lot of provocation for what has happened to her. He then concluded in a manner as though looking for some kind of out, "I don't think she's normal." [She was refused discharge or leave of absence. Later the interviewer talked to her]. *Mrs. Sand:* "If I was an accomplished liar, it would help in cases like that." I asked her how that would have helped. She shrugged and then said, "Oh, if I'd been able to say that I'm feeling fine, going out with my sister, get a job right away, file for divorce—then they would say she knows what she wants to do."

(second discharge conference, 9/17/58)—I asked her if she were expecting any particular things to be brought up at the conference. "Oh, I imagine there'll be questions of how I'll be getting along with my husband, something like that." (How will you answer that?) "That's a good question—I get along with him all right, as long as I let him have his own way. I expect to go to work in 2 or 3 weeks, I think that will help—me, anyway." (How will it help?) "Well, when you are doing clerk typist work—you can't keep your mind on your job and something else at the same time. Housework gives you too much time to think." (What are you afraid that you might think about?) "Oh, if I start on housework—I usually think of something someone has done to me a long time back—and if I keep at it I work myself up into a boiling rage." At which she laughed. . . . *Dr. H.* [First question of the conference]: "Isn't it true that you had an argument with your husband one day last week when you weren't there to meet him?" *Peggy Sand:* "Yes." *Dr. H.:* What do you think you've accomplished in the time you've been here?" *Peggy Sand:* "I've learned to face things more realistically." *Dr. H.:* "What do you mean?" *Peggy Sand:* "Well, before, I was bound and determined to get a divorce—there was nothing else. Now, I'll go back to my husband, I'll get a job. Then, if I decide to get a divorce later, I'll be in a better position. I'll go to work to keep me occupied." *Dr. H.:* "How about the children?" *Peggy Sand:* "I'll be home with them more than I am now—I'd be with them every night." (Indefinite leave of absence).

(third discharge conference, 6/17/59)—Dr. H. agreed to "discharge her, and give a certificate of competence." He then went on, addressing his remarks to the rest of the staff, that there was considerable argument about whether she was psychoneurotic. He then quoted almost verbatim from the report of a prior conference . . . which stated that there was considerable disagreement as to whether or not Mrs. Sand was psychotic, but it was felt that she could best be classified as schizophrenic reaction, chronic, undifferentiated. Dr. H. then commented that this may have been a diagnosis of convenience. I asked her what the discharge will mean to her. . . . "I don't see how it will affect my life one way or another. If you can't lick them, join them, I've quit running." I asked her if she is referring to her marriage, and she said "I suppose so." I asked her what she thought the future of her marriage would be. "I can't say, for the next 12 years at least I expect to stay where I am." I asked why 12 years. "By that time the girls will be pretty well grown—and I'll be older and more set in my ways—too old to change, if I'm not too old already."

Once institutionalized into the marital relationship by the initial hospitalization, marital control was supported by psychiatric through California's now-obsolete conditional discharge provisions. In marriages not in danger of dissolution, the hospitalization episode became integrated into preexisting arenas and patterns of marital conflict. The threat of rehospitalization was used by both spouses as a means of controlling the partner's undesired behavior (see chapter 6). A few of the husbands actually made good on such threats.

Peggy Sand had committed herself to Napa initially on a voluntary basis, a move that Mr. Sand described as "for spite," insisting that there was nothing mentally wrong with her. During one of her weekend home visits, Mrs. Sand went off with a male fellow patient and consummated an extramarital liaison with him. On her return, she was brought up to conference and, though not discharged, was given an indefinite leave of absence. As she was getting ready to leave the state hospital, her husband served her with commitment papers to the county hospital:

On Thursday, she was waiting impatiently for her sister to come up and take her. However, her husband showed at about 2:00. "He asked me if I was leaving that afternoon. I said yes I am. He said, no you're not, I'm having you committed. The papers are on their way up now. I said something to the effect, Do that to me, you might as well kill me, I have nothing to live for. He said he's doing it for my own good, the doctors said I was sick enough to be committed."

Mr. Sand made it clear that his actions were related to her extramarital affair, as punishment and as preventive measure:

Then, fairly early, he mentioned something about going into court on July 1st. I asked him why, and he said in order to commit his wife. He then went on at some length as to why he did this. He said he had thought that she had gone in there just for spite or just to hurt him. He said that she had always talked about committing herself to Napa, but he just didn't pay any attention to this . . . (with considerable vehemence) he said for his wife to have done what she did over the weekend, she must have been sick, or something

wrong in her head. He said to carry on this affair with this man the way sh
did, right in front of the children, and taking one of the daughters down t
meet him downtown—she must have been sick to have done something lik
that. He said that he then started thinking back over a lot of things she ha
done in the past that were odd, and wished that maybe then he could hav
understood it better. He implied that if his wife felt sick enough to comm
herself to Napa, he should have realized this. He told about one time whe
his wife had told the neighbors that she did not have enough money to bu
food. He said with much force that if there was one thing about his family
was that they always had enough food on the table. Sometimes of course hi
wife would foul things up with the money, mishandling it, and then sh
might have difficulty getting the groceries but it was her own fault then. A
such times, he would have to take the money from her and give her a
allowance. He then said to me that he didn't suppose that she had ever tol
me anything about this. He said that he could imagine what she told me
that he (Mr. Sand) was a son-of-a-bitch. Mr. Sand said that she had told him
that, and he assumed that she told that to everyone else. (Mr. Sand told m
about his wife's statement about not having money with a very definit
implication that this was a sign of what he now saw as her sickness).

The themes of control and adequate performance of traditional roles ar
clear in these statements. Peggy Sand had attempted to escape from he
husband's control by running away with another man; Floyd Sand reas-
serted his control through the psychiatric establishment. She accuse
him of inadequate performance in his role as provider, which he claime
was false, while he accused her of incompetence in her sphere o
organizer.

At various times during the twelve years of their marriage, Mrs. Sanc
had attempted to change her situation by leaving Mr. Sand temporaril
and by threatening divorce. Her only arena of control was an attempt t
manipulate their marital future:

He says that he plans to go into business for himself, and will try to work
something out on that, but that's the only things he has planned. I then said
that he does not expect to do anything until his wife decided something.

"She's the one that has to decide—whatever she decides, then that is the way it will have to be—don't have any other choice."

Thus, Mrs. Sand made Mr. Sand experience situational dependence and lack of control, both by mishandling the finances and by rendering the marital future uncertain. She expressed her sense that she lacked alternatives, and described his attempts to regain control of the situation:

I asked if since then she had thought of taking any other steps. She answered sharply "sure, I thought of hitting him on the head with a hammer," but added that she thought of the kids and couldn't do it. She said her husband wants her to go home this weekend and that he also wants her to keep books for him at his new shop (this time the husband wants her under his thumb; she is thinking of leaving and has in the past filed for divorce).

SEPARATION AND HOSPITALIZATION

In cases in which separation was being planned, imagined, or undertaken before hospitalization, the effect of the wife's stay at Napa was to crystallize the decision. The husband either finally left or decided that leaving a sick spouse was out the question. George Yale mentioned separation, but adds that earlier "it would have been a lot easier than now. There's less chance now than at practically any other time." Tim Quinn felt differently:

At some point I said, "And now you definitely want to break up?" He replied loudly and emphatically "Want to! I'm going to break up." I asked when he had reached this decision, and he replied, "I think I can best answer your question this way—I came to this conclusion the day I took her up to (the hospital)—they kind of told me the seriousness of it. And at that time I made up my mind that I'm going to stay with this decision. . . . It would have happened eventually sooner or later anyway. Maybe it just gives me a good excuse. I don't know. When you go through this thing and kind of take a mental inventory—it's at that time that a person throws out all the millstones that are hanging around his neck and gets down to the business of trying to lead as normal a life as possible. She just happens to be the chaff."

Those husbands who saw hospitalization as a barrier to separation were responding to the traditional fifties view of marriage as a binding economic and relational obligation that was even more enforceable in the case of an incompetent spouse than it was in the case of someone "normal." They were also constrained by the mental-health law of the day, which specified that a spouse committed to a mental hospital, since she was legally classified as incompetent, could not be divorced. Husbands who saw hospitalization as an opportunity for separation justified their decision by framing the crisis as the "last straw" in a series of increasingly destructive troubles inflicted on them by their wives.

As indicated earlier, a number of the wives had toyed, from time to time, with the notion of separation and divorce; none felt economically or emotionally able to realize their impulse for independence. However, for those wives—such as Joan Baker—who had negotiated with their husbands over separation for a number of years, hospitalization could and did act as a location (psychological as well as spatial) for the gathering of strength to cope with the decision to separate. Nevertheless it was Arnold who left, not Joan.

Separation changed the dependency dynamics of the relationship. Husbands who wanted to separate from their wives complained about their wives' dependence on them, both financial and emotional, and in effect instructed their wives to become more independent. In addition, men who were contemplating divorce were anxious to deny their wives' mental illness and to have them declared competent.

This pressure toward independence and competence was clearest in the Quinns' relationship. Mr. Quinn came to want a divorce in order to marry another woman once Mrs. Quinn was declared competent and given a final discharge from Napa. He was prepared to continue his economic part of the marital bargain, providing for Mrs. Quinn's financial support, but he was not willing to provide for her emotional dependence any longer. Ruth Quinn reports:

[her sister] told him that when we found an apartment he would have to pay for the apartment and he would also have to figure out what I would need for a month, and he screamed and yelled how much he is paying out now, and he did agree that he would certainly take care of me. To me he was very nice—he said he never shirks his responsibilities.

Instructed throughout her marriage, explicitly and implicitly, to depend on her husband both for financial support and for her sense of self and of purpose, Mrs. Quinn was now expected to change her dependency patterns. She found this difficult:

He just said . . . it was that I have been so dependent upon other people . . . I think he offered me advice, but he didn't tell me how I was going to get myself out of bed in the morning. . . . (Her husband is annoyed because of her dependence on the lawyer and apparently also on her sisters and would like to say that she damn well ought to be able to handle her own affairs). Mrs. Quinn: "It's almost a feeling of, why in the hell, why can't you manage your own affairs—you should."

No longer interested in her mental status for her sake, Mr. Quinn was interested in her mental status from a legal perspective for the sake of his divorce action. This position was in contrast to his earlier insistence on her incompetence. In September 1958 he had said:

"If I ever get married again I hope somebody kicks me in the ass with a big fat boot. It's the worst thing that could happen to anybody. . . . But I've got a pretty good deal. If they get too grabby and want to get married, I just tell them I have to wait for years [until his wife is declared competent and thus eligible to be divorced] and they usually run the other way."

But by February 1959 his position had changed:

In talking . . . Mr. Quinn would get angry, and insist that his wife is competent. 'I know damn well she is competent.' At one point he insisted that I also know that she is competent. I agreed that I thought she was competent. Mr. Quinn also stated that his wife is in pretty good shape, he certainly doesn't see her as any longer mentally ill. All of this is interesting in view of his earlier assertion that his wife was incurably ill, and his pressure to get me and hospital personnel to go along with this idea.

The relationships between marital control and dependence, financial provision and decision making, were played out even in these final legal maneuverings. Ruth Quinn said:

Well, mainly what he was interested in was dissolving the guardianship. Then he had told me before that he wanted a lawyer to see after my interest. He told me he would like to pick someone he knew—that wouldn't charge too much—since he was paying the expenses. So we got up to a lawyer's office and the lawyer explained that the reason the guardianship was drawn up was incompetency. And I said yes, I was a patient at NSH for six months. And he said, "Oh, then it was mental illness"—which sounds better than incompetency. George says I was now competent.

In experiencing his control ever over the steps toward the dissolution of her marriage, Mrs. Quinn feared that she would escape his control while remaining outside his care and protection. Habits of a lifetime are not easily erased:

"And now I am striving for an apartment of my own, and I'm a little afraid that when I get an apartment of my own it will be exactly the same thing." This never quite got clarified, but apparently these feelings are related both to the difficulties of her separation from her husband and children, and also to the fact that she still feels under the control of both her husband and the hospital.

Mothers in the Mental Hospital

From the interview data, the relations of these mothers with their children before, during, and after hospitalization appeared to be far less complex and problematic than the marital relationship. I suspect that this is due in part to cultural taboos about feeling role conflict and trouble regarding motherhood, which are much stronger than those regarding wifehood. The Bay Area interviewers often commented in asides that these women's relationships with their children were not always as untroubled as the women averred; however, there are few direct clues to the nature of such trouble in their lives.

Both the practical and emotional responsibilities of caring for children were a source of stress for these women, in the context of an era in which husbands took no part in child rearing. Joyce Noon said of mothering, "who wants the responsibility . . . I've never heard of anybody liking it. . . . It's a hard job to raise children. The hardest part is that you've got to take responsibility for whatever happens to them." She added in another interview, "All I need is three more children and I'd be back at Napa."

Children were not only a source of emotional labor for the Bay Area women, they were also a source of emotional gratification. Goffman writes of the "pains" of hospitalization, by which he refers mainly to deprivation of the comforts of everyday life—showers, snacks—to which one has become accustomed as an autonomous adult (1961). But included in the pains of hospitalization are those rooted in the historical self and its temporary suspension: in particular for these women, "missing" husband or children, or both. Though sometimes expressed insincerely (at least from the interviewer's perspective) or at least ambivalently, the women referred to the temporary loss of their children as a significant emotional deprivation. Few of the women were able to answer the question, "Do you miss (son)?" like Joyce Noon: "No" (laughing and mildly apologetic) "I don't."

While the women were in the mental hospital, others had to perform their responsibilities of housework and child care. In an era in which such tasks were seen as the proper province of women only, female kin (of the wife or the husband) were, if available, expected to take care of the children and household. Both their absence from their children and the use of substitute caretakers were sources of difficulty for the women.

THE MENTAL PATIENT AS BETRAYER

For the wife and mother, her stay in the mental hospital was at once a welcome respite from roles and responsibilities, and a betrayal of her husband and children. An analysis of the female mental patient as betrayer is, in the patient stage of the moral career, complementary to that of the betrayed mental patient (Goffman 1961; see also Warren 1986). In his classic work on the family and mental hospitalization, Erving Goffman writes of the sense of betrayal experienced by persons who have been lured or coerced into the mental hospital by those closest to them, often wives or husbands (1961; 1971). He analyzes the betrayal funnel by which prepatients pass through the hands of their loved ones into the mental-health system and the resentment the mentally ill person feels at this betrayal. He comments, "The patient . . . is likely to feel betrayed and conspired against; and he may continue to until he is well enough to see that the collusive action was taken in his own best interests" (1971, 383). This commentary on the betrayed mental pa- tient is not linked to gender; but grounded in the historical context of the gender and family-role structures of the fifties, the mental patient became the betrayer. The Bay Area woman felt that she had deserted her family by relinquishing her role responsibilities as wife and—most particularly—mother. The interviewer said of one woman, "She doesn't feel up to taking care of her own children, but wants to get out of the hospital because she can't bear the sense of having abandoned them for 'a soft lick.'" A "soft lick" may be a surprising description of a state mental hospital in 1958. But those wives who did perceive their stay at Napa as a sort of moratorium from role responsibilities also experienced a sense of guilt at their betrayal of their families (see also Sampson et al. 1964).

The wife in the fifties family served both the practical and the emo- tional needs of her husband and children. Her withdrawal from her place in the family to the mental hospital meant that she no longer served them—she had deserted them. The women felt that they had betrayed their children by abandoning them to other, inadequate caretakers. Even when the primary caretaker was the child's own father, the woman was sometimes dismayed. A couple of women expressed fears that their male children were becoming "too like" their husbands during their own absence: Joyce Noon said, "He's (son) getting just like him—he's just a little miniature of Mel you know. He looks just like him, he is beginning to act like him you know. And they're so sure of me, you know. . . . It's just like I'm always there, you know. They go right along and then when something happens I'm always there."

The women experienced severe anxiety about their children's reaction to their hospitalization. They worried about how the children were getting along without their care and about what would happen to their relationship with their children as a consequence of the hospitalization episode:

Ruth Quinn (after a home visit): "The only thing is I felt that the children did sort of look to their father—I could see that they felt that there was something. I think the time has probably come that it will have to be explained to them, because I sensed that they feel there is something different about the relationship. My little boy was very relaxed. He put his arms around me, and he ate the ice cream we had. My little girl didn't eat, and though she was very relaxed and all that I felt there was a little bit of—I don't know what you would call it—but I thought they would be more relaxed if they knew what was going on."

Ruth Quinn was typical in her ambivalent worries about what would happen to the relationship if the children did know about her mental hospitalization and what would happen if they did not know.

A common reaction was a generalized fear of incompetence as a mother, where no such fear had existed before. This anxiety was compounded in those cases in which the women were legally mandated to limit the amount of child care they could perform and instructed to place their children in schools or in the care of relatives for stipulated periods of time. For example, it was stipulated that Mary Yale's daughter Ellen be in school for six months:

I asked her what she made of that stipulation. "Naturally I wondered why
. . . I think it's something of a probation." Pause. "I've always thought I
was a competent mother and Ellen didn't seem disturbed in any way. I don't
know. Is this something generally done when patients leave the hospital?" I
said that I didn't know. I added that the stipulation had affected her feelings
as a mother. She teared slightly. "To have it made a stipulation in your release
kind of worried me a little bit." I said I thought it not surprising that it had
worried her some, but that I did not think she ought to take it as a reflection
on her competence as a mother. "You don't?" (No.) She continued, "I feel I
was a good mother. I had patience. Ellen and I always got along fine. Of
course, there were times when George and I disagreed a lot about her. I don't
think that's abnormal."

What tended to happen when the mother returned from the hospital on
a visit, on a leave, or just after discharge, was a sort of self-fulfilling
prophecy. Because of her apprehensions about the resumption of child
care and the other worries already discussed, the returning mother sometimes behaved with her children in ways "unnatural" for her and them.
Paul Mark said of his wife:

"Through all this [her ten-day leave] she was thrilled to be with the girls
although she didn't show it like a normal mother would." (In what way?)
"She wouldn't let them out of her sight, and she didn't joke and kid with
them like a normal mother would. She did hug them a lot. The children are
children; they like to get out and play. She got the idea she wasn't needed
because the girls didn't spend more time with her."

These mothers, and often both parents, worried about harm coming
to their children, in some genetic or predispositional sense, from schizophrenia; they worried about characterological damage to the children
from exposure to a schizophrenic parent or from feelings of abandonment. Shirley Arlen said, "I thought about my kids. It made me feel so
insecure—if I don't have a home for them pretty soon and take care of
them like a mother should they're going to feel insecure probably for a
long time." They worried about the impact of having a hospitalized

mother on the position of the child in the peer group or school. Paul Mark said, "She thought that she was causing us trouble by being in the hospital; she thinks the girls are being made fun of. I couldn't talk her out of that."

The husbands tended to reinforce these women's anxieties rather than allaying them, since, as has been shown, motherly influence was seen as potent and paramount, for good or ill. Several of the husbands began to monitor their children for signs of emotional trouble. Mr. Noon, for example, said that he was worried about his son because "I believe he was getting mixed up just like his mother." These husbands engaged in various remedial attempts in response to what they perceived as their children's trouble. Mr. Vick said that he intended to keep a close watch on them and to take them to a child-guidance clinic at the first sign of any problems. In a rather contradictory solution to his worries, Mr. Noon encouraged his wife to come home from Napa without leave in order to take care of their son, saying that "I thought if she was home maybe it would help out. It has."

The women's feelings of guilt at betraying their children were very upsetting to them; they felt they were in the position of doing what no mother in the fifties could be imagined doing: abandoning her children. By contrast, the women's sense of betraying their husbands was more grounded in the practical tasks at hand. Since they generally had little emotional communication with their husbands anyway, what these women felt they had deprived their husbands of was household labor:

Rita Vick: "I worry about my kids and about my husband. . . . He's still not working and he has to take care of the kids himself. He doesn't complain, but I know it's hard on a man."

Leo Vick (after a home visit): "She hated to go back . . . she said she was all right now and had to stay home and take care of our two babies and take care of the house—being as I was a man I didn't understand how" (although Mr. Vick was unemployed at the time his female relatives were caring for their children).

Louise Oren: "What bothers me most (about being in the mental hospital)— have him work a hard day—then come home—do washing and ironing— he can't do it like a woman."

Paul Mark: "She thought she is causing trouble for being in the hospital. She thought she is a burden on the family . . . because I'm working so hard. I told her I'm glad to be able to work and take care of the children."

Certain of the patients' delusions might be considered functional adaptations to being an incarcerated housewife. In the face of experiencing guilt at having "betrayed" their families, three of the women experienced delusions that "placed" either their husbands or their children at Napa. Mr. Yale said that his wife consistently mistook a child on the children's ward for their daughter, while the interviewer said of Eve Low that "The children don't look well to her, and she's since 'heard a rumor' that they're on the children's ward at Napa." These delusions maintained a metaphoric connection between the woman's role as patient and her historical self, one that served not only to alleviate her sense of having betrayed her family but also to promote improvement by allaying her anxiety. About a month after the comment noted above, an Eve Low free of delusions said, "I'm so worried about my situation at home, I can't devote myself here in this hospital to getting better, or to relaxing or resting, because I'm too worried about what's happening."

Some of the husbands did not hesitate to validate the women's sense of betrayal. They missed not so much the company of their wives as their wives' support services, lamenting the impact of hospitalization on their work load. These husbands could combat accusations of being a betrayer (Goffman, 1961) by making counter-accusations of the wife's own betrayal in relinquishing her role responsibilities:

Noons, joint: Mr. Noon wants their son to see a neurologist; he says to his wife, "I shouldn't tell you that because you're going to get the bright idea I'm railroading him too. . . . You told me I railroaded you." *Joyce:* "Unh unh, you told me that. . . . You told me not to think you were railroading me or anything. I never thought of it. . . ." *Mel:* "You like it up there." *Joyce:*

"Who'd like to sit up there?" *Mel:* "You. You have no responsibilities, don't have to do nothing, make no decisions."

Similarly, Mr. Sand claimed that his wife had admitted herself to Napa out of spite and that she had betrayed both him and her children by her actions. His wife had her own theory of the grounds of Mr. Sand's sense of betrayal: "In a somewhat unhappy tone, she said about her husband, 'he doesn't miss me, he misses his bed partner, that's all.'"

The Bay Area husbands also felt betrayed by their wives' consumption of family resources during their Napa stay. The husbands' inadequacy as providers and the wives' overspending were highlighted by the mental hospital stay. Not only were most patients billed by the county for the cost of room and board, but the husbands earned less (in lost wages) and paid out more (in additional babysitting and other household expenses) as a direct result of their wives' breakdown. These monetary problems tended, however, to have more interactional significance in the ex-patient stage than in the patient stage of the moral career. It took the rare hardiness of a Floyd Sand to suggest to his wife, newly diagnosed as schizophrenic and hospitalized, that her breakdown was costing him too much.

KIN NETWORKS

One way in which these families' costs were controlled was by the use of unpaid replacement household labor from kin. Although some of the Bay Area families were isolated from kin, others lived close to parents or siblings. Female kin functioned as important resources for child care and housework during the wife's absence from the household. But this solution was not an ideal one because kin—especially mothers—were often implicated in their schizophrenic crises (Sampson et al. 1964). Furthermore, the crisis of hospitalization typically aggravated the woman's difficult relation with her family, a fact that complicated further the negotiation of assistance with child care.

Neither practical nor emotional support from kin was easily accepted by the Bay Area women. Although help with housework and child care might be useful, it could become a form of criticism of the housewife and mother's inadequacy. The Bay Area women saw themselves as closely watched by their families. They felt that their relatives were inappropriately concerned that they might harm the children; indeed, some of the relatives and a few of the husbands expressed just such fears:

Interviewer: "You worried about the children because they were in the care of your wife?" *Mr. Quinn:* "Yeah, sure I did. In the improper care of my wife." *Interviewer:* "How are the kids?" *Mr. Quinn:* "Very good. You know, they haven't even asked about their mother . . . I think they're just happy as hell to get out from under. . . . Doing things they never did before. . . . Somebody who is interested in spending a little time with them, which they never had before. The little girl's learning to sew." I asked Mr. Quinn what he told the children and he replied, "I told them that she was mentally sick and had to go to a mental hospital and she was going to be there a long time. I didn't tell them everything. I gilded the lily a little bit. And I let it go at that. They didn't ask for any further explanation. They knew she was sick. I think they're glad to get rid of her, frankly." I asked how they had reacted during the few weeks before Mrs. Quinn went to the hospital and he replied: "They were pretty nervous—they did talk to me."

Accepting emotional support from kin networks was even more of a double bind for these women. Although kin networks could provide help in times of trouble or company in everyday life, they also appeared to contain many of the sources of the women's troubles. A glance at the women's biographies in appendix A of this book or at the original analysis of their psychiatric histories (Sampson et al. 1964) will give some sense of this. Many of the women remained isolated and unsupported rather than engage in confrontations with their mothers or other relatives, while others accepted the help with ambivalence or rage.

Consigning offspring to the kin network gave rise to problems of trust for the Bay Area inpatients. When the caretaker during hospitalization was the schizophrenic woman's mother, the wife's doubts about her

mother's child-rearing abilities precipitated worries about the adequate
care of her children:

Shirley Arlen: "I don't like the way Jack's being—well I can't say raised, but I
don't like, oh I don't know, it won't be permanent I don't think. My mother's
influence over him. . . ." (What do you think she is doing now that you
don't like?) "Oh, she's just going to make him different from other kids.
Cause she won't allow him to play with other kids, cause they might have a
germ or something."

Kinship support networks functioned much more effectively for the
husbands than for the wives during the crisis of hospitalization. Initially,
hospitalization threw the burden of housework and child care onto the
shoulders of the husband. However, in almost all cases the husband
managed to shift much of the burden to others—generally the female
kin of one or the other spouse, but occasionally a female neighbor, and in
one case a father-in-law: "I then asked [James Arlen] who has been
taking care of the house. He then said that his sister comes over, and sees
that the kids go to school. The oldest girl and he do the housework, and
the sister comes over and cooks." While kin networks were available to
the wives as practical or emotional resources but carried a high emotional
cost, the same was not true for the husbands. They were able to make use
of kin resources both because these networks did not have this emotional
weight for them and because in fifties culture it was almost automatic for
the female kin of males abandoned by their wives to provide "female
role" substitution. Although most of the males were able to find women
to perform some part of the household chores previously performed by
their wives, most were still left with more household work than before.
This inconvenience gave the husbands a strong motivation to regard
their wives as well and able to leave the hospital. As Sheldon Messinger
comments, "In some cases, the husband brought pressure on the hospital for his wife's release at just that point when there was a breakdown
of substitute household arrangements, for example, when the patient's

mother was ill and unable to continue to take care of the children"
(n.d., 44).

Going Home

In the mental hospital of the fifties, patients were continually reminded about going home. They were so reminded not only because role
performance in the hospital served as a reminder of role performance out
of it, nor simply because of their worries about betraying their families.
They were prodded by visits from the family and visits to the family,
both of which were defined by staff as transition events between hospital
and home. Visits from their husbands and other relatives were highly
stressful events, anticipated with emotions ranging from anxiety to
dread to delight. If such visits were skipped, there could be problems of
social control on the ward. The emotion pent up in anticipation of a visit
was expressed in other ways:

Mary Yale: The restraint and seclusions records. . . . The first is January 3:
"Patient become anxious because husband didn't come to see her. Trying to
use telephone and trying to get out of the door when she became resistive
and combative." . . . Belts also on January 9, 4 to 6:30 A.M. (the first of six
restraint episodes from the 3–15 January, 1958).

Even if they occurred on schedule, visits could and did create distress.
Chester Low said, "It appears to me that every time I have gone up to see
her something has happened to her on that day or two days following. I
think you could go ahead and graph this thing."
　　Visits from and to home took on a highly symbolic character for the
patients at Napa, since they portended release from the mental hospital.
As Erving Goffman and others have noted, mental patients who spend a
long time in an institution (or, by analogy, convicts in prison) may

become "institutionalized" or "colonists": they make no moves to leave (1961). Refusing visits from and to home, then, is one way—in a system of graduated release—by which refusal to leave can be symbolically indicated. Both Kate White and Donna Urey were, in the interviewers' opinions, Napa colonists. After almost a year at Napa, Donna Urey refused to cooperate with the predischarge steps of visits from and to home:

"I don't think I'm ready to go home yet." Won't go home on weekends. Described by staff as "regressing . . . absorbed in kitchen work."

Working in Imola Broadcasting System and linen room. Planning to do some modern dance with drama group. Refusal to go on home visits is delaying discharge. She said she decided she wasn't going to return home— she feels she's not ready, her husband feels she is. Old plan to work and support herself has revived. Has answered an ad for a ghost writer for a mechanics magazine.

   The conventional explanation for institutionalism is that it is precipitated by a change in identity from normal to deviant, precipitated both by labeling and by the closure of conventional options. But the experience of the Bay Area women indicates that it may be precisely because there is no change in the self and its role that the individual wishes to remain in the mental hospital (see also Braginsky et al. 1969). Kate White and Donna Urey felt better off in the mental hospital than in their places in the family, so they stayed. But eventually the same coalition of marital and psychiatric authority that had precipitated their hospitalization in the first place forced them out of the hospital and back into the housewife role.
   Donna Urey and Kate White's refusal to take transitional steps toward discharge represents an extreme variant of a more pervasive ambivalence about leaving among the Bay Area women. There were powerful impulses driving them both toward and away from a return to their family roles, since Napa represented both positive and negative alternatives to

life in the traditional family. Thus, most—though not all—of the women felt ambivalent about leaving:

Rita Vick (on home visit): "Really, I feel I should go back but what really stops me is I have mixed emotions about it—undecided feelings. One minute I want to go back, one minute, I don't. And I know financially my husband isn't really about to get anyone to watch the children, so I figure why go back to the hospital. I won't get well there. I may as well stay here. I won't get well here either."

Ambivalence was more often expressed indirectly. Even women such as Joyce Noon, who had vigorously protested her hospitalization throughout her stay, were not wholly committed to returning home. Mrs. Noon described how she had become "used to" the hospital:

"I do like the hospital, if I can't be outside." She said that she would rather be out, but if not then the hospital is OK. "When I first got in, I didn't like it at all, now it's got to be a second home to me. . . . I didn't like anything about it, I didn't like being locked up, I didn't like the routine, I wasn't used to living in—what you call—institution life."

After her discharge conference, the interviewer found her unexcited about release: "I asked her if she knew the results, and she said that she did not. I then told her that . . . she was going out . . . she smiled pleasantly and said, without much feeling, 'That's good.' (I was very much impressed at this point by the apparent apathy and indifference she showed.)"

The apparent ambivalence of mental patients toward release—even some involuntarily committed patients—has been noted elsewhere (Szasz 1976; Warren 1982). In this context it was structured both by the difficulties these women had with the roles and relationships to which they had to return, and by their own sense of trouble. Neither return to the housewife role, nor its impending loss through divorce, as in the case of Ruth Quinn, was a wholly positive prospect for these women:

Ruth Quinn: "Right now I am not ready to go. I'm not well enough. Maybe I'm well enough but I know this is the place to face up to things." I asked her if she feels somewhat afraid about leaving the hospital and she replied: "I'm not afraid to go out, but what frightens me is that I would have to get a job. That's what the other patients told me."

Peggy Sand: I asked her how long she had been in the hospital and she said "two weeks tomorrow." I then asked her what it seemed like to her. "Well, most of the time it's no effort for me to appear cheerful" even though she is "not happy." She did say that it felt good that there was "no one jumping down your throat all the time" and "being sarcastic." She said, "I don't want to stay here all my life—just to regain some measure of self-respect."

What we learn from the Bay Area data is that there are multiple meanings that can be attached to mental hospitalization by patients, and that new meanings develop during the process by which hospitalization intersects with the historical self and current roles and relationships. In the context of gender and the traditional family in the fifties, mental hospitalization had conflicting meanings. One facet of experience—housework on the ward—was at once an aspect of hospital control, maintenance, and routine; a way of keeping busy in the fact of dead time; and a means of retaining the sense of self in a context of role loss. But it is also true that, in the context of mental hospitalization as simply marking time, the hospital's routines and activities sometimes seemed meaningless rather than meaningful. As Joyce Noon said of the purportedly clinical functions of OT: "All you can do is make those darn hot pads—on little looms—and you make hot pads and hot pads and hot pads and they act like it's a great achievement to make a little hot pad . . . it's supposed to be called some kind of therapy, or something. But it's making hot pads." Ultimately, the structure of hospital life echoed the structure of the Bay Area women's marital experiences in its elicitation of dependence and in its infantilization.

CHAPTER 5

Undergoing
Psychiatric Treatment

The treatments given to the Bay Area women during hospitalization were those common to Napa and to state hospitals in general during the 1950s. The women participated in a variety of group activities, from group therapy to occupational therapy, and they received what the original researchers describe as "limited and intermittent drug therapy (as well as hydrotherapy)" mainly for sedative purposes (Sampson et al. 1964, 91). But "in the informal usage of many staff members as well as patients, the word 'treatment' literally and exclusively meant electroshock therapy" (ibid., 13). Ten of the women received ECT, three of whom received the full course of twenty treatments during the initial hospitalization. Two women completed only a couple of the treatments because the ECT left them with fractured vertebrae. Although none of the women received individual psychotherapy while hospitalized, a number of them had received it before or after Napa, or both (ibid., 91).

Medical treatments may be understood from the several perspectives of those participating in them, most generally doctors, patients, and ward staff such as nurses or aides. In psychiatric medicine, doctors understand the meaning of treatments through the medical model, with its theories of etiology, diagnosis, and cure. To staff, treatments often mean the maintenance (or otherwise) of daily routine and order on the wards (Goffman 1961). To patients, the meaning of treatments may not correspond to either of those models, but may contain elements of each, in addition to interpretive features derived from inpatient culture and from individual biography. Thus, as we might expect, the Bay Area patients' interpretation of treatments (especially ECT) reflected their position as women in the traditional family structure of the fifties.

Electroconvulsive Therapy

Since the sixties, the use of ECT on women—in particular on house-wives—has been extensively discussed in the autobiographical ex-patient literature. These accounts stress the frightening and coercive features of the treatment as it was given in the fifties and sixties to female patients. Electroconvulsive therapy was in the fifties, and still is in the eighties, used with greater frequency on women than on men—both the earlier and the later statistics show that about two-thirds of ECT patients are women (Wells 1973; Grosser et al. 1975; Warren 1987a). This disproportionate use has been defended by psychiatrists on the grounds that more women than men are depressed and thus require ECT treatment; it is attacked by feminists and ex-patients as a reflection of combined psychiatric and patriarchical control of women. The feminist criticism of ECT likens it to another phenomenon "discovered" in the seventies, wife battering:

Many husbands beat up their wives. . . . Other husbands just sign consent for the "medical treatment" called shock, and let the experts do it for them. . . . Calling unusual, perhaps troublesome behavior an "illness" allows any woman to be punished with psychiatric imprisonment, shock, psycho-surgery, drugs, branding, loss of credibility. What a convenient way to control housewives who don't live up to the expectations of their husbands. (Bozarth 1976, 27)

If the Bay Area women had refused to consent to ECT, their husbands could have consented for them and thus combined marital with psychiatric control in precisely the manner described by Ollie Mae Bozarth (see also chapter 2). Some of the Bay Area husbands whose wives resisted ECT did in fact sign consent forms, while others did not. Not surprisingly, those women who were forced into the treatment were resentful; however, the overall response to ECT on the part of the Bay Area women varied contextually, both over time and with the woman's place in the traditional family structure.

There was in the fifties (and still is today) considerable disagreement among psychiatrists whether ECT is a useful, benign treatment or a barbaric and damaging one. But both proponents and opponent generally agree (with some very recent dissent) that it has amnesiac side effects. A former president of the American Psychiatric Association refers to the

almost constant impairment of memory that accompanies electroconvulsive therapy. It may vary from a mild tendency to forget names to a severe confusion. . . . At first it tends to cover a long period prior to treatment, then gradually to diminish to events immediately before treatment. It is often distressing to the patient, and may continue to some degree for several weeks or a few months following the termination of treatment. (Kolb 1973, 641)

Experts and informants disagree over whether "full memory finally recurs for all patients, or whether it remains patchy, for at least some patients, in the long term" (ibid., 642). What the medical model classifies as a side effect of ECT was for the Bay Area women its intended effect: loss of memory. Medical treatments, they reasoned, had a purpose; ECT was a medical treatment that made them lose their memory; therefore, memory loss was the purpose of ECT. Their interpretation of ECT focused on the purposes and effects of memory loss in both the patient and the ex-patient phases of the moral career. During the hospital stay, ECT was interpreted in the context of uncertainty and control; on the return home, the focus was on the impact of memory loss and on the restoration of roles and relationships.

There were three general classes of forgetting, which—besides the more general cultural problem of forgetfulness itself—patterned the women's memory loss and had different impacts on their selves and their family interactions. First, they forgot particular people and relationships, including centrally important ones: the existence of husbands and children, and their own place in kin networks (the latter symbolized by forgetting their own names). Second, they forgot routines and events of everyday life, from reading a certain book to how to make cookies. Finally, they forgot what had been troubling them prior to hospitalization.

In the mental hospital, as David Rosenhan (1973), Erving Goffman (1961), and Maurice Temerlin (1968) have shown, staff interpret all patient behavior as symptomatic. The Bay Area data make it clear that the reverse process also occurs: patients interpret all staff behavior as therapeutically intended. Indeed, even mundane activities or events in the hospital were seen as having therapeutic significance. For example, Shirley Arlen told her husband that the radiators knocked at night in her ward in order to test the patients' nerves. As a corollary to this general principle, any and all effects of psychiatric treatment will be interpreted by patients as the intended therapeutic effects (though the psychiatrists distinguish between therapeutic and side effects). Thus, the most commonly experienced side effect of ECT—the temporary erasure of some memories—was construed by the women as the purpose of ECT. For example, Shirley Arlen said:

I think the shock treatments are supposed to make you forget—when you do break down or whatever it is you do to get in here—I mean you're pretty sick and I think shock treatment is to make you forget a lot of things that got you sick and the way you felt and everything like that—I mean it succeeded with me—I can't remember a lot of things—and a lot of people try—try to remember—but I'd rather not. There's some things I'd like to but I think it was for the best that I can't remember a lot of things.

Among those who interpreted ECT as intended to erase their memories of their problems, some, like Shirley Arlen, approved of this idea. Joan Baker, too, wanted to get shock treatment to help her forget, and thus become a "different person":

I asked Mrs. Baker about the idea of getting shock treatments. She said, "I don't care what they do, as long as it helps me—helps me not to be depressed—helps me to be a different person, to like people. I want to forget—I don't know if I can or if I know what I mean when I say it—but my father never liking me as a child made me feel I was a monster, I was different, making me hide in my bedroom."

A number of women, dimly aware that they had said and done embarrassing things in the prehospital phase, were glad to have forgotten the details.

Other patients inclined to the belief that such forgetfulness would do them harm in the long run, by their failing to deal with their problems consciously. Eve Low said:

I did not feel that I wanted shock because I don't think it is to my advantage to forget the incidents that happened to me as a child because it seemed to me that—ah—those incidents that were buried in my subconscious . . . so terribly unpleasant—it caused me to have a complex. . . . Well, after I remembered these different things, it explained to me why I felt as I did.

It is an irony of shock treatment combined with psychotherapy that the one treatment involves an imputed medical authorization to forget while the other involves the injunction to remember. A number of the patients were perplexed about this issue. Mary Yale, for example, had "many questions concerning whether she should think about her troubles and feelings and history (her term: 'analyze'), or forget about them (her term: 'repress')."

In the late fifties (though very rarely in the eighties) state-hospital mental patients could be given ECT without their consent; thus, ECT was experienced as coercive medical control. Eve Low discussed the unpleasant effects of shock and the way in which "forcing" the treatment on her exacerbated her "paranoia": "I don't believe that I can speak as coherently—I don't think my train of thought is as connected. I am more apprehensive. I am more fearful at . . . what will happen to me . . . because . . . until I received shock I had never really been forced to do anything." Like the feminist critics of shock treatment in the sixties and seventies, Eve Low was concerned with the combined impact of medical and spousal authority in her treatment: "She went on to say that she'd been getting shock, though against her wish, and that she feels its purpose is to make her forget things, and to change her attitude, including her resentment at her husband for committing her."

But medical authority has subtle as well as overtly coercive aspects that can lead patients to consent to procedures they might otherwise shun. As Charles Lidz and his colleagues have shown, patients consent to ECT when it is presented to them as a last or sole treatment option, without which they are bound to deteriorate progressively (1984). Some of the Bay Area women, though fearful of ECT, regarded it as a potential panacea simply because it was a medically authorized treatment. The Bay Area women saw it as a form of succor:

Ruth Quinn: Mrs Quinn stated that she is afraid of shock treatment but she feels it has helped her a great deal.

Rita Vick: I asked Mrs. Vick whether she thinks ECT is helping her. She said, "I have noticed some improvement. I can be a little gayer for longer periods."

But in addition to the medical desperation factor, responses to ECT also varied over time with changes in the women's emotional situations and marital relationships. Thus Rita Vick later changed her mind about the value of the treatment: "'I thought the shock treatments would help.' (Have they?) 'I don't know. I don't think so. They made me forget some things, but not enough. I haven't had enough, I guess.' (Are they supposed to make you forget?) 'That's what I heard—that's what everybody tells you—that it's to make you forget.'"

In one unique but interesting case, the physical aspect of ECT as an intervention was taken literally by the patient and translated into delusions about her bodily state. Mary Yale, having experienced ECT as a therapy related to her body, attempted to come to grips, interpretively, with its bodily purpose—since all therapeutic activities, as indicated, "must" have a purpose:

She is trying to understand "intellectually" mental illness and shock treatment . . . (if shock has) changed her physically—not mentally, not in her memory, but physically. . . . At another point in the interview she commanded me to watch her face closely. Did I see anything different? Is her face drawing up? Did I notice her ears moving? And look at her body. . . . She told the charge nurse that she was "all out of shape."

Thus, ECT could feed into delusions and into paranoid feelings of being victimized by conspiracy, by the nature of its administration and its impact on the patient's body and mind.

The self upon which ECT had an impact had not only a contemporary dimension—mental patienthood—but also a historical one. The memory loss attendant on ECT was interpreted by these patients in the context of their social place: the historical self and its network of social relationships, and general cultural values such as the preference for remembering over forgetting. The Bay Area patients' memory losses related to everyday life as well as to their emotional troubles and were integrated into self-conceptions related to personal competence at remembering.

The women were divided on the advisability of forgetting one's difficulties, but uniformly disliked the loss of everyday memory, as well as associated effects such as losing one's train of thought, incoherent speech, or dulled feeling. Donna Urey, two days after her second shock treatment, said, "'Ever since I had that shock I can't even remember reading things.' (How does it feel to suddenly be like this?) 'It feels awful. Because usually I can remember pretty much everything but knowing something and not remembering is pretty terrible.' (When did you first notice it?) 'Right after I got my first shock treatment.'"

Persons may characterize themselves, or be characterized by others, as having "good" or "bad" memoires. Donna Urey characterized herself in the interview above as having a good memory for things she has read, so she was bothered by the ECT-related loss of memory in that area. In another interview, however, she characterized herself as typically forgetful; the ECT loss of memory, therefore, was just another in a series of forgettings that were "shocking" but normal for her:

(How does it feel to have memory sort of—go out on you like this?) "I don't know, it feels shocking—when I was at home—it happened the same way. . . . If I—if the kids don't remind me of something—then I forget—like if their Daddy tells me to phone him at work, during the day, and if they don't remind me than I forget—" . . . (Well you know one thing I would be kind of interested in, is if you could kind of collect your impressions of what it's like to be—to suddenly—have some holes in your memory?) "It's not unusual." (Not unusual for you?) "No."

Since these interviews took place over time, it was possible to trace the patients' changing perspective on the treatment throughout the patient and ex-patient stages. Joan Baker's experience of ECT began with her hope that it would make her into a different person.

(2/25/58): Felt better after ECT, "I wasn't depressed or despondent. . . . Now, I don't feel anything."

(3/4/58): After ten ECT she says that nothing is nearly as important to her as it has been and at no time (in the interview) did she show strong feelings about anything. . . . But she says she dislikes and fears ECT.

(7/31/58) [after release]: "I have trouble remembering stuff. It must be—I've heard that shock treatment will make you forget things."

(9/18/58): She used to worry all the time but now she doesn't. She attributes this change to ECT.

There is evidence from the Bay Area interviews that ECT may function repressively—that is, allow the person to forget disturbing events or persons. Rita Vick, who was an illegitimate child and who had lost custody of six of her eight children, complained, "I can't remember my children's birthdays or my birthday." After a weekend visit that Mr. Yale described as very tense, the interviewer talked to Mary Yale:

I asked very early about her visit home, and she looked puzzled. I recalled that we had talked last week about her plans to visit home, and she couldn't recall this. She stated flatly that she had not been home over the weekend. Later in the interview she was slightly troubled and doubtful over the questions I had raised about the weekend, and was wondering if it was perhaps possible that she had been home. What she did recall of the weekend was a very vivid nightmare, the first since hospitalization.

The patients were sometimes aware that their forgetting was at times repressive. Mary Yale said that she was bothered by her loss of memory because "I want to know why I forget those things."

Troubling persons and relationships commonly forgotten by these women included the existence of their husbands and children, their own names, and the professional nature of their relationship with their psychiatrists. It is conceivable that these women's lapses of memory involved the repression of their resentment at their housewife and mother roles, their sense of isolation and lack of identity, and their sense of the combined medical and marital power that controlled their hospitalization. For example, Eve Low, who had forgotten both the existence of her husband and her own name—at times thinking her name was her mother's, and at times taking on a name unrelated to any kinship or marital ties—said of her delusions:

they seem very real. And yet with the other part of a person's mind—with my mind I suppose that I always knew that it wasn't—yet I guess—I must have wanted to get away from myself and by being someone entirely different, away from my family—by saying I wasn't my mother's child—and also wanted to get away from my husband certainly—because I told you and [the Napa psychiatrist] both that he wasn't really my husband."

In the same vein, two other women refused to tell the Bay Area interviewers, during the initial conversations, whether they were married or not.

In addition to its effect on memory, the clinical literature on ECT's side effects refers to the way in which it can generate either slaphappy or silly feelings on the one hand, or blunted and confused feelings on the other. Both responses were noted by the Bay Area interviewers. Rita Vick was described by the interviewer as having undergone a "remarkable transformation" in that her "depression and ideas of reference were gone" after ECT but also as being in the throes of a "hypomanic euphoria." Similarly, June Mark was described, after ECT, as no longer depressed and "almost compulsively cheerful . . . gay." Both the interviewers and the patients commented on the blunting of feelings that they saw ECT as having caused.

An interview with Rita Vick illustrates the various perceived effects of ECT on memory and emotions and the patient's ambivalent and shifting feelings about the treatment:

She had just received ECT the morning before the interview and she seemed, as she said, "a little woozy." She had some difficulty recalling the events of the weekend. She attributed this to ECT but seemed calmer than she had previously and showed less overt anxiety or tension. She seemed mildly depressed throughout the interview, but at no time did she seem on the verge of tears or express, as she has in all of the past interviews, feelings of complete hopelessness. In spite of all this, she didn't look good to me. She seemed much less alert and more apathetic than formerly, and rarely smiled. . . . Her thinking seemed slower and less clear . . . Mrs. Vick remarked that she seems to feel better since starting shock—she feels more calm. "When someone makes a loud noise I don't jump . . . I know it's a stupid thing to think, but I'm afraid they might hurt my brain some way—that they might affect my brain. But the doctor knows what he's doing."

Forgetting can have a reparative or a disintegrative function. Regressive forgetting may be useful in restoring a person's equilibrium following traumatic experiences. The specific impact of forgetting events in the past depends on the present importance of the events; while forgetting traumatic events may be restorative, forgetting mundane events may be traumatic. As Peter Berger and Hansfried Kellner have pointed out, the reality of everyday life is the bedrock upon which we build our sense of a secure self in the world (1970). Losing touch with everyday life—with a book read, with a church service attended—can threaten that sense. This latter sort of memory lapse was particularly disturbing to the women in the posthospital stage not only because it reflected back to them a culturally incompetent self, but also because it damaged their sense of role competence. A housewife who could not remember how to bake cookies or sew on buttons was, in the fifties, no housewife at all. The women's sense of incompetence, induced in part by the fact of hospitalization and in part by ECT, was magnified in those instances in which the husband had shown himself to be a good "housewife" and child nurturer in her absence.

In individual cases, forgetting details of everyday life could have fateful consequences for everyday life. Prior to hospitalization Shirley Arlen had learned from her mother-in-law that coitus interruptus was not a sensible means of contraception. ECT, however, had erased this knowledge. Soon after she and her husband resumed sexual relations, she spontaneously recalled what she had been told earlier, commenting "I just felt like dying when I remembered it." Again, it is possible that such fateful forgettings are functionally repressive; during the postpatient phase, Mrs. Arlen was trying to convince her unwilling husband that they should have another child.

The effects of ECT on memory and the expectation of memory loss were both at issue in the Bay Area women's relationships—especially their family relationships—in the ex-patient as well as the inpatient phase of the moral career. In addition, ECT-related memory loss was sometimes an issue in the interview situation (see appendix B).

Forgetting persons, which was frequent, seemed to be a truly interactional difficulty; one image that the patient did not want to project was that of a person unable to carry on routine social interaction. This problem was complicated by fears of insulting the other—that the person was not important enough to be remembered. As to the first, it is clear that one function of remembering someone's name is to demonstrate that one has the social competence necessary to participate in an ongoing social relationship: to the other's name are attached items of the common culture. There are probably other devices that people use in an unconcious way that perform this same function, such as recalling an event experienced in common, or making a private joke. Correspondingly, one function of the phenomenon of filling in the other's memories (and the embarrassment of the other when one doesn't fill in) is to aid the forgetter in maintaining a favorable self-image: the image of a competent person.

It appeared to some of the Bay Area interviewers that their respondents used ECT-related memory loss as an excuse to forget. Although it was difficult to document other than through inference, their suspicion was of "purposeful" memory loss and the use of ECT as a rationalizing account:

Donna Urey: Throughout the interview the effects of ECT were marked in her slowed and somewhat thickened, flattened affect, and her mild confusion. She seemed to be discovering her memory loss only as I asked her for information which she could not remember. When, after a while, I switched to inquiries about her family, she brightened and said with comparative enthusiasm (and perhaps relief) "Now that's something I can tell you about!" . . . Although her memory loss is obvious, there were times when I felt that she was helping this along. This was principally when I was probing about her and her husband's feelings about her working.

The context for producing forgetfulness, as indicated by this example, was not wanting to talk about subjects that were painful, embarrassing, or revealing.

This apparently feigned forgetfulness in social interaction in order to avoid interview topics occurs in other social situations. Ex-patients who have had ECT can conveniently "forget" and use ECT as an excuse. Paul Mark described his wife's attempt to avoid involvement in some civil litigation that was unconnected with the hospital episode: "Her sister wants June to be a witness and June said no. Her sister told her that she

might be subpoenaed anyway. . . . June told her that if she was subpoenaed, she would tell them that she had had shock treatment and that
she didn't remember a thing."

The motives of husbands and wives were sometimes at odds on the
subject of memory, with wives wanting to remember and failing to and
husbands wanting them to forget and not reminding them. The outcome of such divergent purposes was conflict over past marital ex-
changes. Thus, ECT-related memory loss became part of the everyday
dynamics of marital interaction for some of the Bay Area families in the
hospital and posthospital phases of the moral career, especially in the first
weeks after release.

Husbands often wished to have their wives forget the emotional
troubles, including marital strife, that had precipitated hospitalization.
Richard Karr commented on his wife's long-term memory loss as proof
of her successful cure by ECT, saying that her memory was still gone,
especially for the period when she fell ill, and that "they did a good job
there." Mr. Karr, like several other husbands, used their wives' memory
loss to establish their own definitions of past situations in the marriage:

Mr. Karr said that Wanda "couldn't remember anything" that happened
after Christmas. He feels this is all for the good. "We (that is mama) have
decided if she remembers what she did OK, but we're not going to tell her."
He doubts (or perhaps I should say he hopes) that she will not remember,
not that she did anything to be ashamed of, of course. But she "wasn't
herself" then.

Other relatives, too, found it in their interest to have the ex-patients
forget; thus, they could freely redefine past situations:

Eve Low: "Now I am sure that my memory (of being molested, as a child, by
my mother's brother) is true, even though my mother, who came down last
week, said that it is all nonsense. However, before we left the house last
Sunday night, she was explaining to [other relatives] why she wanted me up
here, you know, she wants me to have the full treatment she says. I should
think that would entail a great deal more than what I've had apparently, but
she said that she thought it would make me forget all those things. . . . I'm

afraid my mother wants me to have more shock so I'll forget all those things that happened. But I don't want this."

Different relatives had different interests either in recalling incidents forgotten because of ECT, or in collaborating with the patient's forgetfulness.

Wanda Karr: During the post-hospital episode, on the occasion of her mother 'bringing up' embarrassing incidents connected with her psychotic episode, Wanda told her: "Mama, stop telling me those things! I went to the hospital and they made me forget them. Now don't keep bringing them up! You're not doing me any good." When asked if her mother had stopped, Mrs. Karr said, "Well, in her way." Mr. Karr, for his part, expressed pleasure to the research interviewer that electroshock therapy had made his wife forget her hostile outbursts against him in the pre-hospital period.

Mary Yale: She did not recall her pre-hospital delusions of being a homosexual, a man, growing a beard. George reminded her. . . . She told him not to remind her of anything else.

Reminding patients who did not want to be reminded, and not reminding patients who did were both more commonplace than reminding patients of events that did not (in the belief of the teller) ever occur. In fact, I encountered only one such inventive process in the data; in the following account, Mr. Vick had claimed that Rita's mother had come to see her and made terrible accusations against her in the hospital. Rita, however, had no memory of this event, while her mother denied it.

Rita Vick: has told me that she remembers her mother's visit and that her mother did upset her, but doesn't know whether her mother said all those things [her husband] accused her of having said. However, Mr. Vick told me that Rita does not remember the incident at all, and this is why there is all this controversy about whose version of the visit is correct—his or her mother's.

In one family, the forgetfulness attendant upon ECT treatment had a dampening effect on a romance between a Bay Area ex-patient and a male ex-patient. Upon the resumption of their contact in the ex-patient phase of the moral career, they were embarrassed by mutual memory lapses, perhaps as much by their status as reminders than anything else. Ruth Quinn said about the meeting:

It was rather strained at first. I found that there was a great deal he didn't remember. He was in the process of 12 shock treatments when I met him. And when I met him I think I was about two or three weeks off shock. So perhaps I don't remember some of the things that he told me. He didn't remember that I had two children. But he thought I was divorced and was surprised to hear that I'm not divorced.

The original Bay Area researchers noted that ECT can have a positive effect on the restoration of harmonious family relationships once the patient has been restored to the family, describing "the specific effects of electroshock therapy in blurring memories incongruent with the selves the patients and her intimates are reconstituting" (Sampson et al. 1964, 151). But ECT-related memory loss was at times damaging to the emotional ties between family members, most particularly when the patient forgot she had them. Shirley Arlen, admitted for postpartum depression, forgot that she had given birth to her child, who was nine months old at the time she was released to resume care of him. Although she had been reminded by others of his existence, she appeared to have lost her emotional memory of him as her child: "I guess I feel sort of strange with him. In being with him. I don't know, I guess I just feel sort of strange with him. . . . I just don't even feel like he's mine, for some reason. . . . I think he's nine months now . . . I really don't know. I can't even remember when he was born."

ECT also affected marital communication and shared interpretive processes. For some of the couples, ECT provided a convenient rationale for the wife's untoward behavior. For some of the women, the fear of ECT limited communication with their husbands, while for some of the husbands, fear of their wives' reactions hampered the attempt to repair ECT-related memory deficiencies.

Both patients and their husbands made use of ECT to explain away certain types of irregular behavior, including memory loss itself. Family members seemed abnormally aware of memory lapses: not only were memory lapses attributed to ECT that otherwise might have been explained differently (say, tiredness or upset), but many lapses that might otherwise not have been explained at all were remarked and categorized as ECT-related:

Mr. Yale is eager to ask the hospital doctor one question: how long the shock treatment will go on. He has mentioned this on several previous interviews, and the interviewer asks why this particular question is so important. He said it was because of her lack of memory, and "I have the completely unscientific idea that when the shock treatment stops her memory will come back and then she will be well."

Other sorts of undesirable behavior were rationalized by patients or their intimates as a consequence of ECT rather than of renewed emotional disturbance:

Mr. Yale visited Mary on the ward a few days ago and finds her behavior very disturbing. He called his friend . . . tonight and asked him if he thought Mary's reaction was from shock treatment.

Mary Yale: "Some days I'm not functioning well, not thinking clearly. It's not all the time, not every day. Maybe I want to blame it on shock."

The fear of being rehospitalized and receiving ECT against their will affected at least three of the Bay Area patients throughout the decade following their first admission. Instead of communicating disturbing feelings and thoughts to their husbands, these women kept silent for fear of resumed medical–marital control of their lives. June Mark in 1959 commented that "It's nice sometimes to have a shoulder to lean on. But now I don't know if I should with Paul. He thinks right away that maybe I need shock treatment." Mary Yale, in 1972, said that she had "a dread fear of shock" and was afraid to express her feelings to her husband for fear of reprisal in the form of ECT. She added, "shock treatment is a helluva way to treat marital problems—the problems involved both of us."

Marital communication was also affected by ECT the other way around: the husband became extraordinarily careful to treat his wife gently and not do anything to upset her (see chapter 6). Sometimes, this kid-glove approach conflicted with the wife's search for her past. In one ex-patient incident, Rita Vick became angry with her husband and quarreled with him over these tactics:

"I forgot all my children [she names the six of whom she had lost custody] except [the ones she has with her current husband of whom she has custody]. Well, Sunday, I was going through my album and I seen these children, and I asked my husband, 'who are these children? They look so familiar. They ring a bell but I don't know who they are.' So he lied to me and told me they were the children of some friends of ours. So I accepted it and I believed it. I said 'oh.' So I looked at some more pictures and he left the room and went to his mother who was in the other room. And he told her that he lied to me so I wouldn't worry. . . . And I was relaxed. I wasn't thinking about those children or missing them. I understand why he did it but it made me angry when I found out. I kept looking at pictures and then I found a piece of paper which explained all my children. I got very angry . . . I started yelling . . . after he explained I accepted it and forgave him. But now that I remember those children all those worries are back."

The effect of ECT on preexisting marital patterns was that communication between the spouses—already quite restricted in most of these marriages—became further narrowed.

The Bay Area husbands were generally quite favorable to their wives' ECT, though several thought the idea was distasteful and refused to sign consent forms (including one who was in the process of marital separation). The interviews with the husbands contain numerous references to their wives being restored to their old selves by ECT or, alternatively, being transformed into new selves. Mr. Mark, for example, said that after the first shock treatment his wife "seemed improved 50%." Mr.

Vick said that the treatments were "settling her nerves . . . she was pretty calm"; his expectation of the treatment was that it would re-domesticate the family and erase the tension and anger in the relationship: "We would be happy together and bring up the children better. I don't know if that will do it but that's my idea."

Many husbands saw ECT as designed to erase their wives' troubles, including past ventures toward independence or criticism of the marital relationship. As Mr. Karr said of the treatment's purpose, "They're trying to give her a clean mind. A new start." This desire to wipe the slate clean of prehospital difficulties may account (at least in part) for the husband's reluctance to get involved with the wife's attempt to restore her past. Not only can the withholding of information serve as a weapon in marital conflict over the definition of various situations, but it may also provide a way to restore the status quo ante of the traditional family—or perhaps even institute it where there had been a failure of "proper" sex roles from the beginning of the marriage.

It is difficult to assess, in everyday life as opposed to experimental settings, the restoration of memory in ECT patients. The patients in this study were embedded in social networks that included husband, children, and other relatives who could and did fill in gaps for them. Thus, the restoration of memory may be in part—or entirely—a process of relearning, after ECT, under the tutelage of others.

The process of remembering for the Bay Area women was one in which spontaneous recall was supplemented by reminders from family members and others, by learning routines such as cookie baking, and by searches through the environment for clues to the past—as Rita Vick did with her photo album. By the end of the original study, and certainly by the time of the 1972 follow-up, these procedures had resulted in a considerable restoration of the past for these women—with occasional exceptions. In the 1972 interviews a couple of women reported that they did not remember the events immediately surrounding hospitalization, and in one of these cases the ex-patient did not recall her first ECT treatment. But overall, since these women lived in families and had not been subjected (at the time of original study) to the brain-damaging effects of extremely numerous and lengthy ECT series, they were able eventually to reconstruct a sense of their own history and of their roles and relationships within the family.

Other Therapies

For a number of reasons, the other therapies used at Napa State Hospital did not provoke a response comparable to ECT among the Bay Area women. In part, the special peculiarity of ECT (also noted recently in Lidz et al. 1984) is in the absence of any cultural precedent for it. Neither during "normal" medical care nor through exposure to advertisements for over-the-counter medications did anything resembling ECT enter the experience of mental patients. Furthermore, the procedure underlined and symbolized the coalition of marital and medical coercion that structured the woman inpatient's experience in the fifties mental hospital, particularly if it was administered without her consent.

The other therapies, therefore, were subject to interpretation by patients, but were far less controversial. Interestingly, hydrotherapy—applied to at least as many women as ECT—was never discussed in the interviews by any of its recipients. Discussions of group activities or of pill taking by the women were common but not especially detailed. The women varied between seeing these activities as meaningless, as therapeutic, or as features of everyday life on the ward, to be judged accordingly.

INDIVIDUAL AND GROUP THERAPY

As Horwitz (1982b) and others note, lower- to lower-middle-class patients who do not share a common culture and vocabulary with therapeutic professionals may derive little or no benefit from individual therapy. A couple of the Bay Area patients were familiar enough with therapeutic culture to facilitate medical communication—which in practice means that the patient understands psychiatric terminology and accedes to the psychiatrist's attempt to frame her life within it. But other patients had little comprehension of the authoritative meaning of talk therapy and assigned it to their own conceptual categories:

Joyce Noon: (Have you talked with the doctor on the ward?) "I talked to him, but I don't . . . get no satisfaction out of it. I mean the doctor says—he comes in—and I mean there's absolutely nothing to tell—I mean the more he tells the less sense it makes . . . he just came in and sat down and said, ah, who are you?—I said who I was. And, ah, he didn't say anything special—he started to talk about the human nature—and how he was a witch doctor, he was talking about or some sort of thing, and I told him that I—I didn't think it was any of my business, this learning about psychology or human nature. I told him I didn't want to learn anything about it, and he said well all right, and that was the end of that."

Later Joyce Noon seemed to realize what the therapists intended, but wanted no part of it: "You can't get nothing out of a psychologist—nothing! All he wants to know is how you feel."

The talk therapies provided important experiences in analysis and self-reflection. While still hospitalized, the organized talk provided in group therapy helped these women to develop a sense that their lives were not uniquely troubled; that other women, other wives, felt many of the same things they did. In the posthospital stage an irony emerged from this sharing. One of the declared purposes of the mental hospital in the fifties and sixties was to return female patients to their husbands as more "adjusted" wives and mothers. Instead, the very self-analytic and reflective processes encouraged by the hospital enabled female patients, sometimes for the first time, to begin to grasp the structural origins and shared nature of their emotional troubles. Not only some of the wives but some of their husbands began, as a consequence of the social processes of hospitalization, to question the situation of women and the role structure of traditional marriage.

Group activities were sometimes seen as helpful in a mundane sense not intended therapeutically: learning that other people have problems too or feeling less isolated from interactions with others. As Donna Urey commented, in group therapy, "she expressed her feelings and others express theirs. Listening to others helps a great deal." Very occasionally, group or individual talk therapy came to be seen by the Bay Area respondents from within the medical model, as treatments in the sense the activities were intended by medical authorities. Eve Low, describing how her outpatient individual therapy had helped her, said, "I guess it actually is a treatment. I know they used to talk about it but I never used to be able to look at it that way; that is, really a treatment. But I think I know what they mean." And Joan Baker said, "I wonder what else is there to talk about. Then all this stuff pours out. I feel better too, talking about it."

In this predominantly lower-class group, it is not surprising that women who received only group therapy regarded themselves as not having had any treatment at all; as Horwitz (1982b) notes, lower-class psychiatric patients expect physical interventions rather than talk therapy. Joyce Noon, for example, who was recorded as having group therapy, said to the interviewer that "I'm not getting anything—just sitting around," and on another occasion complained that she had had no "physical" or "vaccinations."

Other women found group therapy less than therapeutic. Several complained that they might have been able to talk about their problems individually, but that the group intimidated them. Rita Vick, for example, commented, "They never stop to think that there are some things people can't say with others around. You can't express yourself and say what's bothering you. It's not just me. Other girls tell me the same thing."

Later, Rita described another, rather different problem associated with talk therapy, which a number of other Bay Area patients had also noticed: "They say that's good therapy, to talk about your problems. But it doesn't seem to help me because I can talk about them but darn it I can't seem to find an answer for them." One of the problems with the medical model as a way of interpreting these women's troubles was—and still is—that it focused on the individual, psychological level of analysis to the exclusion of a more structural approach focused on the sociological characteristics of their lives.

PILLS

The Bay Area women were unquestioningly obedient to the Napa psychiatrists' drug therapies, with the exception of Eve Low and Ruth Quinn, whose husbands had both at one time been involved with pharmaceutical work. Eve, who had pressed her psychiatrist unsuccessfully for information on the pills she was given, eventually resorted to keeping them under her tongue, a tactic that was eventually discovered by one of the nurses. Ruth Quinn also attempted to influence the course of her medical care. She told an interviewer, "And I won't take medication. I had asked (the doctor) on Friday if he would take me off—so Sunday I took my last pill. It's been four days and I know very well that when you have been on tranquilizers for several months you are bound not to feel too good."

In the posthospital phase, a few of the other women joined Eve Low and Ruth Quinn in their protest against medication, often because the pills made them feel sleepy or unable to perform their household functions. But during the hospital phase, obedience was the general rule; patients rarely speculated spontaneously in the interviews about the purpose of the pills they took; when asked to speculate, their responses were generally framed as relaxation or a relief from nervousness: Shirley Arlen, when asked what the pills she took were supposed to do, said, "To relax you, and help you to sleep."

This lack of curiosity about the pills was probably related to the cultural familiarity of pill popping as a solution to troubles in our culture, coupled with various structural sources of obedience. There was no organized movement in the fifties, as there is in the eighties, directed at the promotion of informed consent among mental or other inpatients;

the doctor's authority, at that time, was organizationally unchallenged (see the epilogue for a contrast with the early seventies). Furthermore, the social class of most of the Bay Area sample was such as to discourage challenges to medical authority (Horwitz 1982b). These women took their pills obediently because there was no cultural precedent for their not doing so, because they wanted to display a properly obedient attitude to authorities, and because they were willing to take or do anything that would help them to feel better.

In contrast to pill taking, part of the appeal of ECT to those women who found it helpful might have been precisely its cultural unfamiliarity. When medical authorities resort to a procedure as drastic and peculiar as ECT, a signal is given both that there is something very wrong with the patient and that unusual medical measures are being taken to cope with the problem. But without adequate information, even this possible function of shock was problematic for the patient. Rita Vick contrasted pill taking with ECT, underlining its unknown quality: "Sure the pills help. They keep me from getting so nervous or excited. They help. But the shock treatments—I don't know what they are doing for me, if they are helping or not. I'd like to know what it's doing to me but I can't find anybody to give me information."

When women receive a disproportionate share of coercive medical procedures, such as ECT, in a historical context of traditional family and gender roles, the meanings of the treatment come to combine elements of the medical, the marital, and the interactional. ECT, more than the conventional-seeming treatments, affected these women's selves, lives, and marital relationships in far-reaching ways—ways that cut across their various roles and reached from the fifties into the future. The meanings of psychiatric treatment, like the meanings of labeling and mental hospitalization, reverberate, for those affected by them, through time and space, permeating individual biography, family life, and psychiatric history.

The Ex-Patient

CHAPTER 6

Return from the Mental Hospital

With the exception of Donna Urey, all the Bay Area women were discharged from Napa during the three years of the study; all but Ruth Quinn, Joan Baker, and Cora Thorne returned to the families that had precipitated their difficulties in the first place. They were released in accordance with the stipulations of the mental-health laws of the fifties, which required that discharge be a graduated and conditional process.

For mental patients in the fifties, return from the hospital was generally accomplished in a sequence of stages. At first, the patient was not permitted any visitors at all. After certain indicators of "progress" had been established, patients were permitted visits from family members. The next stage was visits home, first of seventy-two hours' duration, usually on weekends, and later ten-day leaves of absence. Patients were generally discharged subject to certain conditions, and into the custody of their next of kin, to be unconditionally discharged only after a further hearing a year later. By the end of the Bay Area study period, fifteen of the patients were conditionally and one (Peggy Sand) was unconditionally discharged, while Donna Urey remained at Napa. These provisions gave the return from the mental hospital certain features. First, transitions were gradual, rather than abrupt, with the special problems and pleasures of the gradual. Second, the provisions of conditional discharge continued the coalition of psychiatric and marital authority that had been established during earlier stages and exacerbated the dependence of the woman on her husband. Third, the bureaucratic stipulation of conditions both provided a context for uncertainty—as bureaucratic stipulations generally do—and allowed considerable room for selective interpretation on the part of the spouses. What they were often particularly concerned to misinterpret were any provisions that cost money or that reminded them of the mental-hospital episode when they wanted to forget it.

The Bay Area ex-patients and their spouses had now to reestablish their marital roles and relationships. The hospital episode was interpreted by most of the respondents as having had beneficial effects on the ex-patient and her marriage: either as a turning point or as a restorer of the traditional family's status quo ante. But at the same time the episode was something to be forgotten, to be put aside, in order to continue everyday life in the marital relationship. The housewife role was pivotal in these processes of restoration and distance. Doing housework successfully functioned for both the husbands and the wives as an index of mental health; conversely, leaving housework undone signaled emotional trouble.

Although all the women returned from the mental hospital, many were again institutionalized, either during the study period or later on (see the epilogue and appendix A). The provisions of conditional discharge allowed a return to the mental hospital to be used as a threat by husbands against wifely misbehavior and, more occasionally, as a threatened retreat by wives from husbandly demands. The initial hospitalization at Napa was not, for the majority of the wives, the end of mental-health treatment.

Reestablishing the Marriage

Reestablishing their marriages was difficult for the spouses at several levels. For almost all the women, leaving the hospital meant a return to being a housewife; for those who were not returning, it meant being cast off from control and dependence into an unknown for which they were neither socialized nor prepared. For some of the women, return was to marriages in which the partners wanted to "try harder" and "make it work," whereas for others it meant return to a still-hostile spouse. For those who were committed to their marriages, one theme of return was that of change: change in the former patient, the husband, or the marriage. The other theme was that of *no* change: what was proposed was the restoration of the state of affairs before trouble began, with a ceremonious burial of the hospital experience.

THE PROMISE OF CHANGE

Cultural notions of hospitalization, especially mental hospitalization, are intertwined with concept of change: change that occurs, first and foremost, in the mental patient, but also in those who surround the ex-patient in primary relationships. Both the mental patients studied by Erving Goffman (1961) and furloughed prisoners "want to feel they will 'make it' because they are now different" (McCarthy 1979, 78). So did the Bay Area women and their husbands.

The wives felt improved by hospitalization in two ways: by the effects of the moratorium and by the effects of the therapy. The attainment of calmness, rest, and relaxation was cited as one of the major benefits of hospitalization. The researchers reported of Ann Rand, "She has felt much better having been hospitalized—she doesn't know how to explain the difference in her feelings before hospitalization (tense) and now (relaxed)—in reactions to flood—it was the flood of '55 that she once said precipitated her troubles." Mrs. Rand, like many of the women, reported that hospitalization had increased her insight into herself and thus her ability to withstand the stress of external events. And Mrs. Karr was among those women who felt transformed through the metamorphosis of her relationship with her mother:

I commented to Wanda, with a question in my voice, that she seemed very different than before she went into the hospital. She said, obviously delighted, did I think so? And that her (husband) had said this to her. I asked her whether she was ever able to express anger at her mother or her parents before she went into the hospital. She said that she had not been able to do it. She said that she often felt angry, but that she was just unable to do anything about it. She commented that even now there are times when she was just unable to do anything about it. She commented that even now there are times when she doesn't say anything although she's very angry. I said it seemed to me that these times were becoming less and less frequent. She agreed. . . . Wanda indicated that before she went into the hospital there were often times when she was very angry indeed at both her step-father and her mother. She went on to suggest that this included her father, too, and that often as a child she was very, very angry . . . previous to the hospital she did express some of it to (husband). Wanda said that she did indeed feel changed, "very different."

In several marriages there was a disparity between the wife's and husband's assessment of her posthospital change. In such marriages, the wife insisted that the hospital had changed her for the better, while the husband disagreed, saying that she was still the "old self" to whom he had objections. In the posthospital stage of the moral career, for example, Rita Vick argued that hospitalization had improved her ability to function on the outside, while Leo Vick insisted that she was as incompetent as ever, within her assigned role of housewife. Mrs. Vick said that her husband kept talking about sending her back to the hospital: "he feels that I am not responsible, that I don't keep the house as other women do, that generally I don't act like other women do."

Spouses promised change as well as the ex-patients. For some of them, the wife's troubles and mental hospitalization were framed as a turning point in the marital relationship—a way out, at least partially, of the marital separateness that had existed prior to Napa. There were a number of areas in which the turning point was proposed: in enhancing communication, redistributing role responsibilities, promoting more mutual rather than separate leisure-time activities, or promising to lessen the isolation of wives whose husbands worked too many hours or who had too many jobs. Several husbands expressed a renewed interest in their wives as persons rather simply as role incumbents.

George Yale: "I am more interested in Mary as an individual than before. . . . I've never seen her as a person other than my wife. . . . She never had a chance to make use of her talents. . . . I think I've been holding her down a lot."

Mel Noon: "I've wised up—never did until she got sick—I never realized—gave it a second thought about her, her feelings—what was going on in her world and mine."

Other husbands focused on the need for household responsibilities to be more equally distributed among wife, husband, and children:

Paul Mark: "I think children should be taught some responsibility. For instance, they shouldn't come home and leave their coats around. I have told them this and I have told them to do things rather than have June doing everything. Some effort on my part and on the kids' part will help." (What was it like before?) "The kids didn't do the dishes or anything, and I didn't! I am from the old school—I figured I was the working man and she was the house lady. So I figured—I was not going to do anything." This was said with a self-punitive tone and with an air of "I will be different from now on."

In their own ways and words, these husbands recognized the structural sources of their wives' discontent in the marital relationship.

But for other husbands and wives the problem was not the position of women in the fifties, but rather the woman's adaptation to it. For these families, the hospital turned the women back toward the traditional housewife role, nipping in the bud the thoughts of independence that seemed to have helped precipitate their current troubles (see chapter 3). Joyce Noon described her turning point: "We'd like to get a new house and start from the beginning . . . I hope I'll be able to be a wife and mother. . . . I wasn't taking care of my family—my husband was doing more than I was—lots of things I should have been doing." Redevotion to their place in life as a consequence of mental hospitalization was expressed in tones of reconciliation or defeated apathy. Mary Yale said, "I was in revolt . . . about leaving home. . . . I know I wasn't taking marriage as seriously as I have since." And Joyce Noon: "I'm married to him and that's all there is to it. He just wants me to do what he wants me to do, that's all. . . . I can't do anything different." Donna Urey saw the Napa experience as reinforcing the pragmatics of her housewife role: "I feel like I've changed a great deal. I've gotten a lot of good pointers. When I go home I'll be able to use those—like new cooking and menus—because I have a big family and have to economize a great deal."

For four of the women who had made vows to return to the traditional housewife role, the symbol of this turning point was pregnancy. One of the four had a miscarriage and one had a child during the study period; others delivered after it was over. Becoming pregnant served the obvious function of reaffirming the traditional gender roles within the family. None of the spouses referred to the tradition-reinforcing functions of the pregnancy and motherhood; but all seemed to be anxiously but happily awaiting the new offspring to bring positive change into the posthospital family situation. Donna Urey, who had spoken of her housewife and mother roles as one source of her troubles in the prehospital phase, remained troubled in many of the same ways; however, expecting her sixth child was a source of hope for the future:

(This was the last interview with Donna Urey, in May 1960; she has just announced her pregnancy to the interviewer): "and they say now you take one project—and your whole house is clean we'll say—which mine never stays that way—"(How does your husband feel you're doing?) "Fine. He says there are times when I get a little upset and I get very over-anxious for things to be just so but he says that can be handled. . . . I would say things are looking rather good, for our side of it. With all these new things happening one right after the other. There for a while things weren't looking so well. But we look at a different point of view and openmindedly we find that it's not so bad after all."

For a few women, hospitalization was a turning point away from some of the elements of the traditional housewife role. The impact of mental hospitalization on these women's consciousness of the limits of their place was somewhat ironic in view of the overt stress in hospital ideology on retooling these women as proper wives and mothers. But the hospital had also provided these women with the opportunity—indeed at times the mandate—to become reflective about their lives and about the sources of their trouble. For some this led to a reevaluation of their roles as housewives and of unsatisfactory relationships in general. Mary Yale, for example, said of housework, "A husband should help. When I get home I will get him more involved." Similarly, although the hospitalization episode reinforced their sense of dependence on the husband for some, other women learned to feel more independent at Napa. Rita Vick said, "This place has made me look at my husband differently. . . . Before I would have been lost without him. I relied too much on him and was afraid to think for myself. Since I came here I feel more . . . independent, less dependent." For some of the wives, mental hospitalization seemed to provide enough of a shock to the marriage to enable previously resisted steps toward independence to be taken. As indicated in chapter 2, Mary Yale and Shirley Arlen began to work outside the home for the first time since marriage, while several women began to take driving lessons or contemplate (none of these plans came to fruition) taking college courses. In at least three other cases ex-patients applied for jobs for which they were turned down; Ann Rand, for example, took a civil-service test for a federal government secretarial job, which she passed, but she had not been contacted about a job by the end of the study period.

But there is a problem with promises of change—or with those changes initiated early in the posthospital stage—they are made within the context of a structure inhospitable to change. As Wanda Karr commented during a posthospital interview she was still "home all the time, in these four walls." Even in the short run, changes in self-knowledge could be undermined by shifting circumstances. And in the long run, there was a tendency for those marital patterns that had existed prior to hospitalization to re-form, and thus for the women's troubles to take the same shape as before:

Ann Rand (almost two years after release): She said Louis was very busy at the shop and was also teaching four nights a week . . . she was frustrated in her present work situation and entrapment in what she considered meaningless work. . . . For her husband, working with his hands . . . all day is satisfactory but she does not want to participate in it. She says that she always thought she wanted to get close to him but not so close that all they ever talked about was furniture. . . . She went on to say that she loved her husband and had no thoughts of getting out of the marriage, which she had at other times, and that he was very kind and very gentle, and a good man in so many ways, but. (But what?) She said her children now were getting older and didn't need her around the house and she said she would just go off her trolley staying home alone all day but on the other hand she did not want to work down at the furniture shop all day either. . . . I asked her if she was feeling exploited by her husband as this had been one of her concerns before hospitalization. She denied that she felt exploited and said yes, she had felt that way before but not this time. Somebody in the hospital had told him that she needed to feel needed by him and his way of doing this was to have her work for him. If she ever protested he would generally say, "it's good for you" . . . and then she said, "Oh, am I going to be one of those kinds of women who are never satisfied? Louis is a wonderful man and everyone says he is. But I don't dare make any critical remarks about him around relatives or any of the neighbors. You are the only one I have ever said anything to. And, really, I should be thankful—he's kind and he's a good father and I have a nice house." . . . I think it was right in here that the telephone rang. . . . "Well, she said, I just talked to Louis and told him I wanted to quit working in the shop after I get out of here and I want to become a vocational nurse. And he got very upset by this and said that if I did that he would give up the shop and just teach."

It is not easy to change deep social structures with flimsy resolutions. Husbands drifted back to working at night or to separate involvements; housework returned to the provenance of the woman; communication, so hopefully begun, closed back into separate worlds. Wives once again became disenchanted with the household role or lost the sense that their discontent was legitimate. As the 1972 reinterviews demonstrate, while many of the spouses were divorced or separated over the intervening years, very few attributed any permanent, positive change in their marital relationships to the stay at Napa. Even before the termination of the 1957–1961 interviews, the sense of a turning point was beginning to die in most—but not all—of these marriages. Traditional structures of dependence and control, based as they are in fundamental economic inequality, are not promising locations for the generation of more equal, satisfying marriages.

DENIAL OF CHANGE

For some of the families, the women's release from the hospital meant a return to the status quo ante and a denial of the hospital experience. The denial of change was particularly common among the husbands. Especially in the first stages of the posthospital relationship, before some of the conflicts had resurfaced, the Bay Area husbands seemed to have a vested interest in insisting that "nothing unusual was happening" with their wives—better put, perhaps, nothing unusual *dared* happen.

Mr. Yale: (How are things going?) "About the same. Nothing spectacular or different. Normal. Medium." . . . Says that Mary sees friends less often than before she was hospitalized "but it doesn't have to do with that. It's because I'm so busy, and her working. . . . I don't know if I'm just more reluctant to talk about things or that there's nothing to talk about. I have my mind on so many damn things . . . family life isn't a problem right now and so many other problems. We had a crisis at one time and that was the main problem to get over and through. I'm pretty involved now in union things, contract things, and so on. . . . I'd rather not talk about anything that happened seven months ago. That's all past. (Shoving away gesture with arms and hands.) Done. Mary feels the same way about it. We're done with it. Everything that happened then is over."

A number of wives, too, focused their posthospital release adjustment around an attempt at restoring prior roles, often within the context of a "honeymoon" period of renewing their relationship.

Mrs. Mark commented, "I'm so happy to be home." I observed that she certainly looked happy. . . . "I am so happy just to be here just puttering around." The adjustment she achieved prior to her release is maintained. There is a denial of all that is disharmonious and she gives the appearance of working at being cheerful and at having 'good' feelings toward her husband and children. The fragility of this adjustment is suggested by a number of things: her fear of being perceived as complaining about anything. Her defensive reactions to her husband's teasing. On one occasion, for example, he jokingly said with reference to his guitar playing, "June is my best critic." Mrs. Mark responded anxiously, "Oh, I'm not critical." . . . Her underlying ambivalence and her fear that this may be revealed is illustrated by another incident that occurred when I was leaving. Mrs. Mark playfully poked Mr. Mark in the ribs and said teasingly, "I'll beat you up." In a jocular manner—although with some annoyance—Mr. Mark responded "Oh yeah? It won't be a real beating up because I will let you do it." I jokingly said, "I will leave before all this starts." Mrs. Mark immediately approached me and said, "Oh, I didn't mean it." I responded immediately and said, "I know, I was kidding too." . . . When I asked her what she had been doing, she answered, "Just puttering around the house." Mr. Mark commented, "She's been cleaning. There were a lot of things in the house that I didn't take care of while she was gone." Mrs. Mark anxiously interjected, "Oh, I didn't say that." . . . Her disappointment with her position in life is focused upon her financial situation and is probably related to her ambivalence toward her husband . . . revealed in the following ways . . . "I'm so happy to be here even in my little house . . . the roof leaks but I don't care."

To forget about the mental hospital was impossible for these couples in the face of reminders of it; thus, those who attempted to restore the status quo ante tried to erase any reminders. First, the respondents distanced themselves from the hospital. Second, they underlined their current normality by restricting interaction with persons who reminded them of the mental hospital. And finally, the passing of time provided an element of distance.

Moving house sometimes functioned as a way of distancing the family from associations with Napa; a few of the respondents directly linked their moving plans with this escape theme. In another place—out of the area, city, or even state—the couple could "begin again" and would not have to encounter hospital personnel, outpatient services, or neighbors who were aware of the wife's breakdown in the first place. For a number of these families, such trouble was seen as a close proximity of the wife's mother or mother-in-law (see also Sampson et al. 1964); the escape was not necessarily from the hospital experience but from the locus of those troubles perceived as causing the wife's breakdown in the first place.

(While on a visit to the hospital Mr. Yale reported that): Mary said that she wanted to move away, and specifically, away from her family, her mother. . . . Mr. Yale is for this; he concurs with her feeling that "If she ever comes back to the house it will be the same thing all over again, she'll be back in the hospital."

(After Mary's discharge): Mary has, according to Mr. Yale, changed her mind this week about moving. "There is no good running," she said to him and he agrees, but he holds, "a change of environment isn't running, and "might be good." Mr. Yale seems to be futurizing his plans: "I've always wanted when I finished my schooling to move out of the Bay Area—out of the state."

George Yale: The house is still for sale. . . . When I entered Mr. Yale was sitting looking at some maps . . . he said that . . . they were planning to take a vacation. . . . He said he guessed they would go to Oklahoma.

Distancing oneself from an experience such as Napa is a matter of relationships as well as geography. Barbara Laslett and myself note that one method of distancing is the restriction of interaction to those who will support attempts to regain a sense of normalcy (1975). This process, referred to as "quarantining," has two dimensions: restricting interaction with others who remind one of the experience, where such restriction is practicable; and restricting involvement of those others with the inner self when it is not practicable to restrict involvement altogether.

Getting out of the house and visiting with friends and neighbors is a type of interaction that underlines normality; it is a normal type of association with normal types of persons. Associating with relatives and friends who were aware of the mental illness and who might refer to it and look for ongoing signs of trouble was seen by the Bay Area wives as involuntary, though perhaps requiring an inner, defensive distancing process. But there were, in the ex-patient phase, certain persons who, by virtue of the types of interaction one had with them, underlined abnormality: the researchers in the Bay Area study, fellow patients, ex-patients, and psychiatric workers.

The interviewers noticed that conversations with them became more restricted as the patient moved out of the hospital and through the posthospital phase (see appendix B and Sampson et al. 1964). Similarly, although a few of the women associated with ex-patients, none kept up the contacts with hospital friends that had been anticipated prior to release and none joined ex-patient organizations. In a joint interview, the Yales made the following remarks: "People often say that they will come back to the hospital but they don't. They probably want to forget." Mr. Yale wanted Mary to join [an ex-patient organization] and she said, with some feeling, "I have more of a desire to be with normal people." Mr. Yale said, "They're normal aren't they?" She replied, "I don't know if they are." Those few wives who did keep some contact with fellow patients tended to do so in a way that preserved their own ego distance from the status of mental patient. For example, in her posthospital relationship with Sylvia, a former fellow patient, Mrs. Rand took on the role of adviser and protector rather than peer to her.

The husbands tended to be even more reluctant than their wives to encourage the women's contact with former fellow patients or with current patients. Understandably, this was most true in cases, such as that of Mrs. Sand, in which the woman became involved in a romantic relationship with a man during her hospital stay. But it was also true in the sense of an indirect, as well as a direct, threat to the marital relationship and to the ex-patient's fragile sense of mental health. Ann Rand "wants to call up (two female patients) when they are back in the community, but Louis does not want her to continue any contacts with them. He does not want her to talk about her hospital experiences with friends."

During the leave-of-absence period, Napa required patients to keep in touch with social workers from the hospital. Those wives and husbands who sought to return to the status quo ante were particularly concerned to avoid such contacts. Since a shroud of confusion usually surrounded the conditions of discharge and the proposed initiation and frequency of contacts with the social worker, there was considerable room for evasive maneuvering on the part of spouses. The Karrs, for example, "misunderstood" the role of the social worker in the context of wanting to "forget," describing her as a "bill collector."

A minority of the Bay Area women, however, did receive follow-up outpatient treatment either at a public clinic or from a private practitioner, though some of the ex-patients who started private therapy had to terminate it after a short time for financial reasons. The step of obtaining outpatient treatment for the wife was taken by those couples for whom the wife's recovery seemed ambiguous and for whom the potential for further emotional trouble outweighed the reminder involved in seeking additional help. One interviewer summarizes a meeting with both Marks:

When I was going to leave Mr. Mark suddenly offered the following information. Mrs. Mark is going to visit Dr. M next week. This is the psychiatrist whom Mrs. Mark saw prior to hospitalization. A social worker at the hospital had told Mrs. Mark that it would be advisable to see a psychiatrist regularly in order to obtain Sparine. . . . Dr. M will decide on Tuesday how frequently he will see Mrs. Mark. She commented, "I hope not too often. We don't have the loot."

But, in general, ex-patients attempting to quarantine themselves do not want the follow-up services of social workers or psychiatrists. Patients with a stake in seeing themselves as mentally well preferred, if possible, not to associate with mental-health professionals at all. The researchers reported, "Kate White saw no reason why the social worker should be that interested right away and felt trapped in a position wherein her role was that of a mental patient and, thus, she was required to tell all and hide nothing." Similarly, they found that "Mary Yale decided she did not want to go to the clinic. She's kind of leery about anything that reminds her of the hospital." Furthermore, the conditional discharge provisions were often described—and resented—as a form of probation or parole: Louise Oren said, "I don't like going there. I just feel like I'm on probation for a jail sentence."

Peter Berger and Thomas Luckman note that one of the ways in which a conception of self, newly developed and fragile, is solidified is through conversation (1967). Conversion and conversation are similar words; conversation upholds the new self. Wives who wanted to see themselves, in the overall sense, as well, restricted those types of conversations that reminded them of their hospital stay or their mental illness:

Mr. Yale suggested, and Mary agreed, that it is more comfortable to be with people who talk about the experience openly than people who avoid it. But Mary qualified this. It was easy to talk with the Smiths because they talked about it for a few minutes, and then you know it was over, and it wouldn't come up again. But with the Joneses there was no mention of the hospital and they probably will talk about it sometime. Mary Yale said: "I'm prejudiced . . . I think it helps to talk to people who haven't—who don't always think of the psychological implications of everything." (To George) "I think we do too much of that, don't you?" He said he did not. "I feel this (psychological implications) discussion is an indication that I'm not quite well."

The internal conversation of analyzing and thinking was also subject to censure as a reminder of the schizophrenic episode. As an interviewer said of Wanda Karr and many of the other patients: "A basic theme . . . concerns 'gaining perspective' on her problems by not taking them too seriously, not 'dwelling' on problems, losing self in objective activities, etc. The counterpoint theme, remembering what went wrong, or not understanding it, and thus remaining vulnerable to further trouble." The instruction not to think or analyze too much was associated with the women's housewife role, as a doer of things and a feeler of feelings for others, rather than for herself. The instruction to think and analyze was, by contrast, an outcome of the hospitalization experience, with its stress on a reflective search for the historical origins of emotional trouble.

In the ex-patient stage, the psychoanalytic strategy was more acceptable to the wives than it was to the husbands. Some of the wives had come to believe that if they analyzed and talked about their problems, there was an increased chance of overcoming them. Thinking, from this perspective, was a curative activity; as Ruth Quinn remarked, "Until I went in the hospital I have never been analytical like I am now. The reason I do it is because I think that if I can understand why I became mentally ill, I might be able to accept it and face reality better."

The husbands, by contrast, were more generally concerned to distance the mental hospital and deny the possibility of further trouble. They also tended to believe that these analytic activities had precipitated mental troubles in the first place and would cause their recurrence. And since in many cases the wife's troubles had been precipitated by her place in the traditional family, any analysis of her situation would be dangerous to her once back in that place. Thus, while the husbands had a vested interest in their wives' not thinking about their marriages or their life in general, the wives had the sense that their troubles were intimately linked with facets of their familial situation and that this connection needed to be brought to light. Like Mr. James, the husbands recommended keeping busy rather than dwelling on their situation: "I think if she isn't feeling well a vacation would do more harm than good. Because she won't be doing anything—she would just lay around the beach and think. . . . I think all she would want to do would be to think about herself, and she wouldn't have anything to keep her busy." The injunction to think or not to think became part of the process of family conflict. One researcher noted of Wanda Karr: "She mentioned that she was interested in her prehospital behavior and often asked husband about it. He said that Mama told him not to tell her. 'She wants—well—it's something like packing clothes in a suitcase or something, hiding it.' Wanda doesn't agree with this [hiding problems] and presses her husband for details."

Although the alignment was usually by gender, perspectives on thinking versus doing were sometimes reversed. Fearful of what their internal conversations might reveal, some of the wives preferred not to "think too much." Once reestablished, for these women, daily life had about it a sense of the precarious and precious. Thinking too much, overanalyzing, could precipitate a return to the troubles that had led to Napa weeks or months earlier. And some of the husbands who had placed their faith in the psychotherapeutic approach to mental illness wanted their wives to continue the analytic process in order to get better. But for those who wanted distance from Napa, it was important to restrict internal conversation as much as interaction with fellow patients and persistent interviewers, or other reminders.

Finally, the passage of time itself distanced the current self and marital relationship from the mental hospital, whatever the intentions of the ex-patients or their husbands. For those wives and husbands who wanted to forget, the passage of time was welcomed as it removed from them the conditional discharge provisions, and eventually even some of the memories of Napa. For those wives who had been ambivalent or who had wished to return, the passage of time also helped erase such feelings. And with the memories of Napa, for certain women, went some of the memories of those troubles that had brought them to the mental hospital. Louise Oren, discussing other people's treatment of her as still sick, said, "I don't let stuff like that bother me any more. That's because it's been so long since I was in the hospital."

Return to the Housewife Role

There are many ironies embedded in the posthospital return to the housewife role. Although housework was a source of strain, trouble, and discontent, it was also a symbol of identity and a grounding upon which to base a sense of the solidity of everyday life. And in addition to the stressful aspect of housework (see chapter 2), there are circumstances under which the everyday life of the housewife may be seen as reassuring. Both during home visits and in the first weeks after discharge, the women reported that they did very little at home besides their old routine activities, and that they enjoyed "relaxing at home": when Donna Urey was asked what she had done on her leave, she replied, "Well, uh, getting back into my routine, as usual. We didn't do anything exciting."

Since the women's identities were embedded in the housewife role, their sense of personal restoration was grounded in their competence as wives and mothers. Restoring a sense of role competence is perhaps best served by the relative incompetence of role substitutes during the wife's absence, and worst served when the spouse or role substitutes have functioned as well as or better than the spouse. Women who could make their household "better" on their return from hospitalization contributed to their own sense of competence. An interviewer reports: "I commented that [Ann Rand] had a very attractive son. She said in a rather sarcastic way, in return, 'you should have seen them when I came home from the hospital. They had not had their hair cut for a month.' . . . I also noticed that the house was considerably more straightened up than when I had been there before." In contrast, Paul Mark commented, "June told me I was doing an awfully good job with the idea that she was not needed here. I told her that children need a mother's love, and that nothing can replace that." Wives who could, like Ann Rand, occupy themselves with cleaning up the residual mess left by their absence could in this way restore their own sense of identity through competent role performance. On the other hand, any residual weakness or strain left by the hospital experience could be exacerbated by immediately plunging into the full round of wifely and child-care obligations. This was one of the many posthospital junctures at which the same facet of her environment did the ex-patient both a service and a disservice. Another difficulty for the women was that (perhaps because of ECT, see chapter 5) they were no longer accustomed to the housewife role within the family. Immediately after their return home the women felt strange and alien in their own place. June Mark commented, somewhat metaphorically, "so many things were changed after I got out of hospital. It was like learning everything all over again. My education, my vocabulary, my English . . . everything all over again. And when I got out of the hospital, I felt weak. I felt like I could have stayed in for a year."

A sense of shock accompanied the inability to accomplish routines in the normal way; many of the women's first efforts in the home were directed toward retransforming routines from the strange into the once-more familiar:

June Mark: Mrs. Mark told me with some concern that, although she is enjoying things at home, "I'm kind of slow. I have to get organized. I have to learn the children's schedules again. It seems like I have been away so long. I guess I am not organized yet." She added that the reason she is slow is because Mr. Mark is at home (unemployed). "We always end up on that couch . . . watching TV." She commented later, "well, it's always harder to get things done with a man around the house."

During the posthospital phase, both the husbands and the wives were concerned continually over whether the wife was getting better or getting worse. For both husbands and wives, the primary indicator of the wife's current condition was her successful performance of the housewife role. Other less central, but still significant, indicators included her role performance in other areas (such as sociability) and her internal emotional state while living out roles and relationships.

For the wives, both the competent accomplishment of wife and mother roles and the experience of proper motivation in doing them were signs of improvement. Adequate performance of daily routines helped them feel they were getting better, which decreased the fear of relapse. Daily routines in and of themselves reassured the ex-patients that they were out of the hospital and to some degree restored to normal living. Conversely, nonperformance or incompetent performance implied decline. Rita Vick said, "I didn't particularly care to get up. I was depressed when I awoke because I didn't sleep very good that night. I didn't do anything that night. I didn't do one thing hardly. I took care of the kids and made the meal and was in such a mood that I didn't straighten out the house."

The same roster of role performances was also used by the husbands (and sometimes by other relatives) in their assessment of the wives' condition. Housework was of considerable significance for the wives; for the husbands, it had perhaps more importance than any other factor in assessing their wives' condition. Doing routine household tasks adequately was a sign of getting better; doing more household tasks than before hospitalization, or doing them better, was an even surer sign.

Chester Low: "Things just seem to be going along fine. She gets the housework done and even has time to herself in the afternoon." He expressed his discomfort "when she got vague . . . she's rational though, she got supper last night."

George Yale: "I told him [psychiatrist] that the difference between now and when she first went in there is miraculous. . . . She had the house all cleaned up, and did the ironing, and had the clothes washed. You might say she was getting back into the swing of things."

When household tasks were neglected or badly performed, this was a sign of their wives' worsening; both husbands and wives spoke as if there were some optimum quantity of time to be spent in household tasks, as well as some optimum performance level, beyond which suspicions of pathology might creep in.

While the performance of housework and child care assumed great importance in family assessment of the women's mental state, getting out of the house and engaging in outside sociability also assumed some importance. Both husbands and wives produced instances of such activities as indicators of getting better and of not getting out or socializing as indicators of getting worse. Richard Karr complained, "She takes care of the children but she just sort of sits around and is depressed because of staying too much around; we didn't go out enough. And thinking too much."

There was a built-in contradiction in the meaning of housework for the Bay Area women. Housework was on the one hand a source of strain, trouble, and mental illness, and on the other a source of reassurance in the restoration to prehospital roles. It is not surprising, therefore, that while the adept performance of housework was welcomed wholeheartedly by the husbands as a sign of improvement, it was regarded with more ambivalence by the wives.

Return to the Mental Hospital

Five of the women were rehospitalized at a psychiatric facility during the period of the research, and many more followed during subsequent months and years (see appendix A). While two of the rehospitalized women were returned from conditional discharge as a form of punishment by their husbands, the others returned voluntarily or were taken back by reluctant husbands in the face of escalating troubles. Still other wives relapsed into symptomatic behavior but were treated on an outpatient basis rather than returned to Napa.

In addition to occasions of return, threats of return were used by both husbands and wives—but more consequentially husbands—as part of their marital control repertoire. Under the conditional discharge provisions, husbands were requested to return their charges to Napa at the first sign of trouble. For Floyd Sand, as we have seen, the first sign of trouble was his wife's affair with another man, to which he responded by having her recommitted. The Noons had an argument while Joyce was on an unauthorized absence (an overlong home visit) and Mr. Noon had her taken back as an escapee. Joyce said, "He sent me back just because I can't get along with him." Other husbands threatened rehospitalization but did not carry out their threats, since the threat itself was usually enough to bring their wives' behavior back into line (see chapter 2). Only one wife, Ann Rand, consistently used the same sort of control tactic as the husbands. She threatened repeatedly to return to Napa if her husband did not meet her needs, having experienced hospitalization as a means of controlling his response to her. She said that she regarded her hospitalization as a kind of victory over Louis in that he became nicer to her and paid more attention to her.

Despite their threats, most of the husbands did not want their wives returned to the mental hospital. The husbands who were fond of their wives did not want to lose their company, but even those husbands who had no such feelings did not want to lose their services. So they insisted, in the posthospital phase, that their wives were well and could function as housewives: the researchers reported of Chester Low that he "does not want his wife rehospitalized because it was just a lot of work and added responsibility that you don't usually consider." George Yale said, "Her return has made my life a hell of a lot easier, she makes the meals, takes care of the kids."

The more powerful person in a relationship may deny that trouble exists rather than label the trouble as mental illness, if denial more closely serves his interests. Such denial can have a negative effect on the mental health of the dependent individual. Some of the Bay Area women felt emotionally distressed in the ex-patient phase; their husbands' denial of their difficulties was an additional strain on them, rather than (as labeling theory implies) a liberation from the self-fulfilling prophecy. First, denial further underlined the women's perceptions that their husbands did not attend to their needs or see them as persons. Second, denial frustrated both emotional and practical needs: the need to be relieved of some household responsibilities and the need to be the object, rather than the subject, of emotional labor. Eve Low, for example, frequently reiterated a desire to return to the mental hospital and a wish to continue to deal with the emotional roots of her current troubles. Her husband just as frequently denied the possibility of further trouble or need for help. In separate interviews, Chester Low commented, "It's all over as far as the family is concerned. It's such a relief to have Eve home that we don't talk much about it"; while Eve Low said, "I don't talk to him much about it [the hospitalization and her continued problems] because I upset him when I do . . . because he said that everything is all right." Eve stressed not only the continued psychodynamic sources of her difficulties, but also her continued isolation in the housewife role: "My mental illness came to a head and led me to the hospital while I was alone so much—I am now more anxious about being alone than I ever was before. I'm anxious now because I'm afraid that I might become ill again."

As in the prepatient phase of the moral career, some husbands did not notice that their wives felt, once again, emotionally troubled. After his wife's release from an earlier hospitalization, Mr. White said, "She seemed to do well for a short time. She resumed her housework and child care without any particular difficulties." Later, he discovered that his wife, without telling him, had been returning to see the psychiatrist. Other wives wanted to return to Napa but did not discuss it with their husbands because they felt that by so doing they would once again betray their families. They felt blocked in seeking help by the family's lack of money or alternative household labor resources, even when the husband was cooperative:

Rose Price is thinking about going back to the hospital. (Why?) "I feel more relaxed there—it's not so tense. I don't know if it's because there are others there like me. And I feel sometimes like I would like to get away from it all." (Do you want to go back?) "Yes, because I need help." . . . But she "can't because we need money for a babysitter. He [husband] would like me to go back. . . . I haven't had a tantrum or thrown anything for quite a while" . . . but she felt "depressed. I worry a lot when I'm depressed. I just seem to incline more to myself."

One ex-patient, June Mark, relapsed to the extent of seeking an ECT series on an outpatient basis. This episode is instructive for what it tells us about the efficacy of various posthospital adaptations in the long term. Initially the couple moved house to distance themselves from Mrs. Mark's mother, who had come to be defined, during hospitalization, as the source of June's emotional distress. Later:

June Mark (5/1/59): I asked her whether she is still seeing Dr. M [outpatient psychiatrist] and she responded "Yeah. Only about every six or seven weeks. That's about all." She quickly changed the subject. "I want to do a lot with the house. I don't know how the wallpaper would look here."

(10/5/59): Mrs. Mark has had another relapse; she is currently undergoing another course of outpatient shock treatments with Dr. M. This will be her third course of ECT. Her concrete, perseverative conversation today is obviously related to the effects of shock. I learned little of the circumstances of her relapse and infer it only from the fact of her treatment. She pointed out anxiously that it wasn't that she was "ready for the hospital again." She told me that the shock is "relaxing" and she needs a "rest."

During this relapse, moving house again was proposed as a remedy for her current troubles:

Shortly after my arrival, Mrs. Mark told me excitedly that she and her husband have recently come to a decision to sell their house. She went on at great length justifying the decision . . . it seemed clear to me that his decision results from Mrs. Mark's recent troubles. This move holds the hope of her relief at being able to leave the neighborhood . . . (also) Clearly Mrs. Mark wants her daughters to grow up in a middle class neighborhood. . . . As I drove away, she called out that she had learned her lesson and would never again have a nervous breakdown.

Again, however, this maneuver was psychiatrically ineffective:

(1/18/60): This was my last interview with Mrs. Mark. I last saw her three months ago. . . . Mrs. Mark seemed pleased to see me. . . . Mrs. Mark told me with a brave, tired smile—that she is about to begin another course of shock treatment. On her last visit to Dr. M—one week ago—she had spoken to him of how she felt people ridiculed her. Dr. M said that this is not true and prescribed more shock treatment. Mrs. Mark feels lost and betrayed. She feels Dr. M and her husband have formed a coalition to force her into more ECT at the threat of rehospitalization. More important, perhaps, Dr. M's reaction has cast further doubt on whether she is sane. . . .

She feels (her ideas) are true but Dr. M told her they are not and her husband backs him up. She keeps repeating "I'm so confused. I just don't know." Then she would add, "I didn't know why people are doing this to me. . . . And then there are things on television. People calling me an 'it.' Like I'm a creature."

So, in many ways most of the couples came full circle during the ex-patient phase of the moral career. Although lasting changes were made in the lives of some, such as the Arlens in the short term and Kate White in the long term (see epilogue), those promises of change that heralded the women's return home proved substantially empty. Only those women who had been removed forcibly from the traditional family, with its obdurate structures, escaped an ultimate reabsorption. It is difficult, perhaps impossible, to change social situations if the proposed change flies in the face of the historical structure of those situations. For the Bay Area women to become more independent in the context of a relation of control and dependence, or to become less lonely in the context of an isolated existence, was ultimately just too difficult. For some, the answer was a return to the mental hospital. For others, it was a recommitment to their lives as housewives and an attempt to forget the pain.

CHAPTER 7

Psychiatry
and Everyday Life

The transformation of the Bay Area women's troubles into psychiatric symptomatology had an impact both on the marital relationship and on the theories used by the respondents to understand and explain their experiences in the world. This impact extended from the hospital into the posthospital phase of the psychiatric career. Once accepted as a way of interpreting the Bay Area women's experiences, the medical model expanded, for some of these families, into more generalized interpretive work. Both husbands and wives added psychiatry to their repertoire of explanatory schemas, proposing mental illness as an explanation for the behavior of others within their social circles. Furthermore, two of the husbands became interested in the psychiatric view of their wives' behavior to such an extent that they began to function as quasi-psychiatrists busy with their wives' "cases."

The medical model came to have a certain authority in their lives both because it was associated with the authority of medicine and because it functioned as a source of assistance in a situation of otherwise intolerable crisis. But in the ex-patient stage of the moral career it sometimes came to be associated with the renewal of trouble, the disintegration of family life, and stigma. Thus, continued acceptance of the medical versus the everyday interpretation of the Bay Area women's conduct depended on the husbands' situated interests at hand, on their wives' moods and feelings (Thoits 1985), and on the use of alternative pathologizing frameworks (such as alcoholism). Spouses who wanted to frame wifely conduct as normal rather than abnormal used a variety of strategies to repudiate the schizophrenic label, from redefining the hospitalization episode as one of physical illness to blaming others for the sequence of troubles that led up to it.

Psychiatric Symptoms
and Everyday Experience

Persons labeled as schizophrenic are liable to a radical questioning of the entire scope of their everyday lives; the depth and breadth of the mental-illness label calls everything into question. Thus, the Bay Area women and their husbands, even after the wives' discharge from Napa, were confused about whether any subsequent troubles were symptoms of illness or everyday problems; they even had doubts about the basic quality of the self (see chapter 8). Neither the women themselves nor their husbands were certain of the ordinary grounds of everyday experience; in Erving Goffman's terms, the woman's place in the familial ordering of things had become dis-ordered (1971).

In the posthospital phase of the moral career, a crucial question for the women and their husbands was whether their everyday behavior was pathological or normal—in particular of any sorts of trouble, and most particularly the sorts of trouble that had previously been defined as symptomatic. The women were unsure whether the difficulties they were having, for example, in doing housework were caused by personality flaws or by mental illness. Shirley Arlen among those women who wondered whether she was mentally ill, or just lazy: "I'm trying to see if it isn't that I'm just lazy. . . . I don't like cooking . . . I don't like to shop."

Curiously enough, one centrally reassuring factor was the fact of mental hospitalization itself; it could be, and was, seen as such a disruptive factor that normal behavior could not really be expected immediately after release. Mrs. Quinn, for example, interpreted her posthospital loneliness not as a pathological but as a "normal" response to her husband's abandonment, seeking authority for such an interpretation in a mental-health pamphlet: "A book for families of the mentally ill—it gives the information and guidance that relatives need before, during and after hospitalization. That book I would like to get. . . . I think that it might be helpful . . . that some of the things that are happening to me now are very normal things."

At the same time, the very experience of hospitalization was abnormalizing, in that it had set authoritative seal on the woman as pathological, or at the very least fragile. Shirley Arlen said that on home visits she just "lays down" to avoid being made nervous by the conflicts between her parents-in-law. She said: "I'm scared to do anything more. I'll just get worse. I don't want to feel any worse so I figure . . . the best thing to do is lay down."

Many of the women reported feeling radically disoriented by the experience of mental illness and mental hospitalization; this disorientation was then interpreted as further evidence of abnormality. The women's confusion about pathology and normality was exacerbated, in some cases, by the memory loss resulting from ECT. As indicated in earlier chapters, the husbands' pathologizing of their wives' behavior in the posthospital stage was grounded in family role allocation and in the emotional condition of the marital relationship. But there remained— for the husbands as well as the wives—the everyday problem of distinguishing hallucinations and delusions from real events and from "imagination," and paranoia from persecution.

HALLUCINATIONS AND DELUSIONS

During hospitalization, the patients' beliefs about the nature of everyday life underwent psychiatric reinterpretation. "Obviously" delusional—culturally implausible—beliefs were discarded as symptomatic. In the early weeks of her stay at Napa, for example, Eve Low exhibited the grandiose delusions typical of paranoid schizophrenics: "if this case [her commitment] is not settled, it will eventually perhaps become a grand jury matter. It will become a trial. I will either have a legal trial or become obliterated, one or the other." Some months later, however, she referred to these beliefs as her "former delusions" and as "ridiculously" grandiose: explaining why she had been afraid to tell the interviewer various things, she said, "being a paranoid with delusions and persecutions and so I was afraid to tell you. . . . I had delusions of grandeur, I was so important, imagine!"

Several of the ex-patients who had earlier been delusional or hallucinating once again heard voices or believed (in one example) that the TV was broadcasting messages specifically for them. The crucial difference in the ex-patient phase, however, was their at least partial acceptance of the psychiatric perspective: that the voices or beliefs were not grounded in the shared reality of everyday life. Eve Low expressed the institutional necessity for accepting the psychiatric point of view at her diagnostic conference:

She then went on at length about arsenic poisoning, apparently talking about a child of hers; she thought that this child was showing symptoms of arsenic poisoning, which Eve said that she had had as a child herself. However, she did not want to tell that to the doctor she talked to because then they would say that she had "delusions of persecution." (Eve was quite pleasant in talking about this, almost sweet. When she said delusions of persecution, she smiled knowingly and everyone else did too.)

Donna Urey learned during the first week of hospitalization to understand her voices in psychiatric terms:

"I started hearing these delusions after my first two children—before my first two children were born." (What were the voices that you heard?) "Well they were mostly—like I told everybody else, these voices are like guardian angels, steering me away." (Can you remember what you were steered away from?) "Well, mostly from distrust . . . mostly I think it was because I was lonely for Albert."

But in an interview about five months after discharge from Napa, Donna Urey indicated a return to everyday or normalized conceptions of voices ("everyone . . . has run across the same thing")—an interpretive feat clearly unshared by the interviewer:

(How about the voices? How have they been doing?) "Oh, I just glide along with them so far as they are concerned." (Is this the same situation—you hear them but you don't pay much attention to them?) "Well, it's this way. If it's good, then there is some sense to it, but if it isn't, then there's no sense to it. . . . Ordinarily what the voices are, is just common sense, and that's of conscience and everyone I know sometime in their life has run across the same thing." . . . (Could you tell me what the voices say, either say or said?) "Well there are times when they have said, 'we're here to help you,' and uh, 'you'll be with us, and if you do that you won't' and that's the time when I think a lot of people really have to use their conscience."

The interpretation and reinterpretation of delusions and hallucinations as psychiatric symptoms or as aspects of everyday life had both a "natural history" and a situational aspect. To some degree the imposition of the medical model during hospitalization propelled the respondents along the path of progressive psychiatrization; and this tendency was partially reversed, as indicated below, by the neutralizing work of the posthospital phase. But moods and situations also played a part.

The husbands, along with the wives, were faced in the posthospital phase with the problem of interpreting the essential nature of the women's troubles. Indeed, this task was legally mandated; as indicated in chapter 6, the husbands—as their wives' legal guardians—were instructed to take them back to Napa at the "first sign" of renewed mental-illness symptoms. This instruction sometimes did, and sometimes did not, fit with the husbands' particular interests at hand. Thus, troublesome beliefs might be interpreted by husbands on the one hand as a renewal of hallucinations or delusions, or on the other as real events.

Once the wives had been diagnosed and hospitalized, it became more difficult for the husbands to believe implausibilities. The husbands no longer sought diligently for sources of hallucinations in real life (such as the "echoing from the street" voices of Mr. Urey), or believed—at least easily—the wife's version of quasi-plausible events. Instead, the woman's hallucinations and delusions were either discounted or dismissed in everyday terms as instances of "imagination": a researcher records, "Chester Low reports that his wife has the delusion that some of the patients are being tested for nursing ability; 'she's not herself, I just let it go by.' He refers to her delusions as 'imagination.'" Indeed, "imagination" functioned throughout the moral career as a way in which implausible perceptions and beliefs were discounted by the husbands. Regarding Joan Baker's belief that people were in their house at night, Arnold Baker said:

"It's her imagination. She has always had a strong imagination. Some people have a fear of the dark and other people have a fear to be alone." . . . He said she was restless at night and tosses and turns, and to prove to her that nobody was in the room he would tell her to get up and turn the light on. . . . She said there was definitely someone bothering her.

PARANOIA AND CONSPIRACIES

Unlike some of the other classic symptoms, paranoia has become a subject for sociological as well as psychological analysis. This is perhaps because the notion upon which paranoia is based—that of a conspiracy of others against the paranoid—is a highly interactive one, amenable to sociological as well as to psychological investigation. After all, conspiracies do exist.

In his work on cycles of paranoia, Edwin Lemert asserts that the person diagnosed as paranoid is typically reacting to something real in the environment, rather than internally fabricating others' conspiratorial behavior (1962). He claims that others' reactions to the troubles experienced by a prepatient (or someone showing paranoid symptoms who never becomes a patient) lead to her redefinition as someone unpredictable, troublesome, or difficult. During this stage of the paranoid cycle, others collude to exclude the prepatient from normal social relations.

In organizations, a real conspiracy against the paranoid person may then emerge, with coworkers attempting to close him off from communications, power, or even the job itself (Lemert 1962). In the family, this cycle takes the form of a betrayal funnel (Goffman 1961). In both cases, the prepatient is correctly experiencing cues from the environment either that others are defining and treating her differently or that they are conspiring against her. What makes the paranoid reaction psychiatrically rather than routinely interpreted is the grandiose expansion of the paranoid claim beyond the actual clues or the actual conspiracy.

The purely psychiatric interpretation of paranoia implies that the only cues and conspiracies to which the paranoid is reacting are generated by internal processes (Cameron 1943). The purely sociological interpretation—which was developed in analyzing the social situation of gay people—implies that the only cues and conspiracies to which the person fearful of persecution is reacting are external, stigmatizing ones (Lyman and Scott 1970; Warren 1974). The Bay Area interviews suggest, with Lemert (1962), that the person labeled paranoid may, under specific familial and organizational conditions, be responding both to symptomatic and to everyday life contingencies.

Several of the Bay Area patients were diagnosed as paranoid schizophrenics or had paranoid beliefs, including Eve Low, Mary Yale, and Kate White. What they claimed as conspiracies in the prepatient stage had been authoritatively dismissed as paranoia in the patient stage. While not all patients are willing to give up their conspiracy theories, these patients did. But in the ex-patient stage, as social critics of the mental hospital, these women came to recognize the operation of real conspiracies against them in the procedures that led up to hospitalization.

As a patient, Eve Low told a delusional tale of how she had been railroaded into Napa by being duped into signing her own commitment papers: "I had been hypnotized . . . at least three weeks before I was committed . . . and I understand that . . . I signed the [commitment] petition under the guise of a fireman coming to my door stating he was a Democrat and asked that I sign for the firemen in Berkeley to receive higher wages." Later she described a more grounded conspiracy:

"I waited there in the hospital to sign myself in—the nurse came with a sheet and I said can I not sign myself in, and she just said no. And as I told you before I felt, well, I'm not going to make a fuss because if I do they'll think I'm mentally ill, so I didn't, and I went into the ward very agreeably. My husband didn't hold my hand—didn't kiss me or anything to say. . . . He's very loving now—and was later. But that was the time when he should have . . . so after I thought, 'what have I done,' because I began to worry about my children. . . . and then, when I was not allowed to sign myself in—I thought 'this is some kind of a trap'—true I was mentally ill, but this just goes to show how something like that can make one more mentally ill."

It is clear from these comments that the experience of betrayal by intimates, the lack of information coupled with arbitrary medical authority in the mental hospital of the fifties, and the fears and terrors associated with the hospitalization process can exacerbate paranoia.

The expansionary potential of paranoia is increased by the experience of hospitalization as a conspiracy. One result is that experiences and persons encountered in the hospital themselves become part of the paranoid's theories instead of those theories being, so to speak, left at the door of the hospital. What could conceivably be a moratorium from paranoia as well as from role stress becomes, instead, an exacerbation of it:

Eve Low: "I was not allowed to sign myself in—in my mind when I was having persecution complexes anyway this just was the ultimate persecution and I was—my wild feelings that I thought I was trapped—and purposely put in there for some ulterior reason . . . [hospitalization procedures] fed these delusions rapaciously. . . . because I had the beginning of a persecution delusion . . . in the fact that I was put in the hospital, not allowed to sign myself in, not given one single treatment or tablet, nobody said 'are you sleeping?' or anything to me from the time I went in until I left—I naturally thought well this is done purposely, here I am—I'm getting worse, nobody's helping me, so naturally . . . where I was having delusions then naturally I had more delusions because I thought well I was really— being persecuted. And you can understand why, can you not. . . . if patients on coming in could have some sort of an orientation—I'm sure it would make a terrific difference because—most people I think—even though mentally ill—they can be reached."

THE PSYCHIATRIZATION OF EVERYDAY LIFE

Interpretive schemes may be produced by special circumstances, but they need not stay confined to them. The use of psychiatric concepts to interpret the Bay Area women's troubles, authorized by medical science and consolidated through hospitalization, was, for some of the respondents, generalized to other people and to other sets of troubles. If psychiatric explanations for personal and social life proved useful or satisfying in one context, then they might prove so in others. Furthermore, a number of the husbands began to expand their role to encompass medical as well as marital dominance.

The husbands in particular began to utilize the "sick" label to explain the conduct of others in the environment of whose behavior they disapproved. To see someone as crazy became yet another way in which that person could be discounted; indeed, husbands used the label on those—often in-laws—with whom they had relations of hostility. Chester Low said, "One of her sisters will become a candidate for Napa if she doesn't cut out her thinking [about Eve's hospitalization]." With the exception of Mr. White, the husbands refrained from extending the psychiatric framework to their own actions and feelings.

Similarly, a number of the husbands expanded the notion of controlling others through hospitalizing them to encompass more than their wives. If mental hospitalization works as a temporary solution to marital difficulties, then there might be an opportunity for similar solutions to difficulties with others.

The expansion of these interpretations and techniques was exemplified by Mel Noon, who according to his wife had been seeking medical explanations and solutions for his problems with his son and his in-laws since her hospitalization:

Joyce Noon: "We went over to the doctor here, and he couldn't find anything the matter with [son]. He even told [husband] so. Still, he's going to say yes there is. He knows more than the doctor. . . . He's worse than an old grandmother, picking at any old thing." (So you have had your fill of Mel?)

"Oh yeah. Everybody has. My family is sick of him. And now he is going to throw my mother in—until he bumps up against my father there." (He's going to throw your mother in?) "Yeah. He's going to have her put away and then he's going to see if he could have my sister put away. That's his idea."

The women, too, expanded the net of psychiatric interpretation to include the conduct of others, though (at least in the interviews) they did not propose involuntarily committing these others:

Kate White commented upon her increased awareness of her father's social isolation and preoccupation at times. She wondered whether he was mentally ill. Her husband couldn't buy this at all.

Rita Vick: "truthfully deep down I think my mother is mentally ill . . . she acts like it . . . now that I look back on it."

Joyce Noon: She described her husband as being sick himself, that he admitted this . . . he was also plotting to hospitalize her mother and her sister.

Sometimes even the teachers of the psychiatric perspective had their lessons turned against them. Eve Low, referring to her outpatient psychiatrist, remarked, "I think he's emotionally mixed up—kind of repressing something—or maybe he is kind of hostile."

A second feature of the psychiatrization of everyday life was the husband's assuming responsibility for psychiatric monitoring. Several of the husbands, as hospitalization progressed, began to cast themselves as psychiatric experts. Mr. Noon, for example, stated that in his search for the causes of his wife's illness "I'm trying to make myself into a psychiatrist. Figure things out." Mr. Vick, similarly, told an interviewer that "he feels it is important to 'understand her case' and in order to do so he is trying to get as much information as possible. He then mentioned the fact that he had gone . . . to talk to his wife's family about her 'history.'" In commenting on his own outpatient therapy, Mr. Vick contrasted it with the research interview, saying "Oh that. . . . It's a different thing. With her [the outpatient social worker] we work on me, but with you we work on Rita." And he formed a coalition with the Napa staff to "work on her" moods and role performances through ECT:

the social worker . . . told me that after she got shock treatment she would be the kind of person she should have been all along . . . happy and calm . . . close to me . . . and . . . a considerate mother and wife. . . . I have seen that she is that kind of person deep down . . . I got her convinced that she ought to take them in order to feel well . . . I told her she would be an altogether different person, that she would be happy, well, she would enjoy life, she would have no more tension.

Acting as a research psychiatrist or aide served as a mode of adaptation to the situation for these husbands. Instead of feeling helpless, useless, or uninformed in the face of their wives' mental illness, these husbands took action. As Mr. Vick said in a letter to his wife, "you are sick now and I will see you get well and then we'll start enjoying our life together." The interviewer commented, "Mr Vick deals with the situation by gathering information for what he perceives as use by the hospital in his wife's 'case' as he calls it . . . especially about her family of origin, and 'handling' her."

Marriage and the
Interpretation of Trouble

The use of alternate interpretive frameworks varies with context—in this case, the traditional marital relationship. In the posthospital phase, the Bay Area respondents planned to have their marriages changed, restored, or dissolved; psychiatric and everyday interpretations of trouble were crucial elements in these processes. Certain consequences flow from interpretive work; for example, Mr. Quinn insisted that his wife was "crazy" while he wanted to remain free from marital involvement, then reversed himself to insist that she was "normal" once he had decided to remarry. For those spouses who did not separate during the hospitalization crisis, both the medical and the everyday model could be invoked restoratively.

Accepting a psychiatric model of individuals and their conduct depends on many factors; within the family, these include the spouses' intentions toward the marriage and the extent of what Erving Goffman calls the "havoc" wreaked by the prepatient's symptoms (1971). Packaging distress neatly into the medical model may serve to reassure the patient and her family that the difficulties they are experiencing can be understood and controlled. Applying medical terms and theories sets the interpretation of what might otherwise be chaotic and inexplicable havoc within a familiar framework, and even promises—at least initially—a cure. As Rita Vick said about her bizarre behavior, "my husband bought me that house . . . and I made him sell it and the furniture and everything. And the second home we bought I did the same thing. But I think [my mother-in-law] kind of understands now, because Leo told her the psychiatrist told him it was my condition that made me do these things."

The psychiatric framework relieved marital crisis in a number of other ways. Since mental illness is an individual problem, the woman's troubles could be reframed as emanating not from her social situation—her marriage—but from herself. And, furthermore, it was not her essential self that was responsible for her bizarre conduct but, rather, a curable—if somewhat mysterious—disease. As Mr. Price said of his wife: "I'll stick with her as long as she needs me, after that it will be no problem." This means he will stick with her until she is well, after which they will get along fine. "Because any act that she can pull now it will be just absolutely from the state of mind that she is in. It wouldn't be anything actually that she would want."

With its provision of the sick and caretaker roles, the psychiatric interpretation of troubled conduct relieved, at least temporarily, the role strain typical in these fifties marriages. For a short while, the wives could rest and relax in the mental hospital, then come home to a period of recuperation and lesser—though gradually increasing—housewife role demands.

While mental hospitalization promotes seeing everyday life in psychiatric terms, it is also clear that there is a tendency running counter to psychiatrization: attempting various sorts of denial of mental illness. This counter-tendency was common among those families most interested in reestablishing the status quo ante, who did not want to change role structures, even temporarily. And, more generally, since mental illness is a discrediting condition, interviews focused on mental illness may be expected to generate neutralizing accounts. After hospitalization, some of the Bay Area respondents sought to retain or restore everyday-life frameworks for the interpretation of their troubles, both by telling posthospital "sad tales" and by shifting the blame for troubles from the ex-patient to someone else.

SAD TALES

The Bay Area patients, like Goffman's (1961) inmates, proffered sad tales to account for their presence in the mental hospital in terms other than psychiatric ones. The content of these sad tales varied, depending on whether they were told during the patient or the ex-patient stage of the moral career. Quite common in the patient stage was the railroading tale (like Eve Low's, given earlier), by which the women attributed their hospitalization not to their own mental illness but to betrayal by others—usually their husbands. Goffman has described the way in which initial accusations of railroading become tempered, in the family context, over time (1961). A number of the Bay Area wives came, in the later patient or the ex-patient stage of the moral career, to reinterpret their husbands' betrayal as "in their best interests."

Wanda Karr: She mentioned asking [husband] about who called the psychiatrist. At first he refused to tell her, saying "Mama said you shouldn't know.

You'd hold it against us." She debated this with [husband], holding that she had needed help, and it was silly to think she would hold it against them. Who knows, she said, what she might have done if they had let it go on. She might have gotten violent she said, set fire to the house, or even killed the babies. She wouldn't have gotten better, that she knew.

Ruth Quinn: "Momma is trying to blame [husband] for putting me in here" (Mrs Quinn laughed at this notion as though trying to convince me that it's an absurd idea). "Both of them are wrong—Momma and [husband]. It's my childhood. Because I'm the one that's in here and I'm the one that doesn't think it's such a cross to bear. I wish that people wouldn't feel that way—I wish that they would understand that one out of 10 will be mentally ill."

Interestingly, these posthospital reinterpretive activities function in the opposite direction from the in-hospital sad tale: they return the explanation of trouble to psychiatry from the world of everyday life. A woman who presents herself as having been "railroaded" by her husband into the mental hospital denies her mental-illness label. If she later changes her tale to one of her husband's activities in her own interest, then by so doing she transforms herself into what others "knew" she was all along: a schizophrenic. These fluctuations of psychiatric and situational self-labelling express the difficulties the Bay Area women faced: if they denied their schizophrenia, then they blamed their husbands. If they denied their husbands' betrayal, then they had to accept the schizophrenia.

Sad tales told by the inpatient are typically tales told by the self (Goffman 1961). It is clear, however, that other people may have an interest in purifying the moral self of the patient (or inmate) and thus may proffer sad tales on her behalf. Typically, sad talers are either professionals paid to do the job (for example, probation officers; see Corry 1984) or family members seeking to preserve the integrity of the self and its place (for example battered wives; see Ferraro and Johnson, 1983).

Thus, not only the wives but also the husbands sought to account for the former patient's Napa stay in ways that neutralized the mental-illness label. Neutralization involved classifying troubles as something other than symptoms: as personality traits, as a normal response to abnormal circumstances, as an instance of some form of pathology other than mental illness, and as physical rather than mental symptoms. Those husbands who wanted their wives restored permanently to the housewife role—and those couples who sought to forget the entire Napa experience—commonly neutralized psychiatric interpretations, with their stigma and implication of recurrence.

Troubles may be framed or reframed as instances of personal foibles. Behavior that could have been interpreted as symptomatic was explained as an expression of traits the woman had always had. Richard Karr said of Wanda, "she's been pretty irritated lately. . . . The weather is mostly what's doing it." He added that Wanda is depressed once in a while, but "everyone gets depressed once in a while." Wanda said that her depression "comes and goes, but I've always been that way though."

Persons whose interpretive work has in the past been guided by some clear and consistent ideology are liable to neutralize psychiatric definitions by incorporating them into preexisting categories. In the Bay Area sample, for instance, Ruth Quinn sought to frame her troubles as alcoholism rather than mental illness:

"I'm an alcoholic and I don't understand why I'm not in the alcoholic ward instead of in the mentally ill ward. . . . I consider myself an alcoholic— that's very important to me . . . I know what I am. That's why I was in the AA. I wanted so desperately to go on living with my husband that I couldn't eat and couldn't sleep and ended up here."

Even well into hospitalization a few of the patients or their husbands refused to acknowledge the "mental" aspect of the woman's illness. These respondents stressed the physiological bases of their difficulties and saw Napa as a general hospital, a form of denial that continued in some cases through the patient and ex-patient phases. Soon after Rose Price's rapid discharge from Napa her husband decided that any future remedial care would be sought from a chiropractor rather than a psychiatrist, and that the psychiatric handling of her problems had been an error:

Prices (joint): Mrs Price said it was her teeth that had been bothering her and she needed six pulled. . . . Mr Price said that was not what was the trouble but that she had nerve pressure at the base of the skull. That was what the chiropractor found out. . . . Mr Price said that they should never have gone to see the psychiatrist but they are on the right track now.

Physical-illness interpretations included a remarkable assortment of ailments:

Leo Vick: "She needs something for her glands . . . she would be troubled by constipation and forgetfulness . . . of course she's not insane, I know that." . . . [asked what insane meant] he thought about this a moment and then mentioned venereal disease. . . . "However with Rita she suffered from a deficiency. And the symptoms of it were that she craved sweet stuff, everything would turn to fat, and she would have trouble remembering. She would also be constipated." . . . Rita herself claimed that she was in the hospital because of a sore back, and that the mental hospital was a general hospital.

Joyce Noon says that "90%" of the patients at Napa are suffering from "epilepsy" and "it's very rare that you ever find anybody there with anything mentally wrong with them."

Wanda Karr: She said that she had been somewhere else before coming to [Napa] (she had been at the County Hospital). She "thought" that she had been in a "gymnasium." She said that they had given her pills at the gymnasium, just like the pills she got here. . . . I asked if there were any doctors at the gymnasium. This seemed to strike Wanda as strange, and she said "Maybe it was considered as a hospital, but it wasn't a hospital."

Since these ex-patients were women, gender stereotypes about the psychological effects of women's physiological conditions also came into play. Menstruation, menopause, and childbirth were all cited either as alternatives to the psychiatric interpretation of their troubles or as having precipitated emotional difficulties:

Ralph James: "Irene hasn't been so well again . . . just about a week now . . . She just started her period a little more frequently and got worse again. It all seems to be tied together, but which causes which I don't know. I was wondering if it was the change of life that's causing it. . . . I have a feeling that a lot is physical that is causing the nervous phase of it."

Another gender stereotype involved in the neutralization of psychiatry was the notion of "episodes." Like the "overactive imagination" used to explain hallucinations and delusions, "episodes" were mysterious—but ultimately nonserious—features of women's lives in the fifties, reminiscent of the "vapors" of the heroines of nineteenth-century novels. A number of the Bay Area husbands were content to frame their wives' past troubles as "episodes" that had been blown out of proportion by psychiatric hospitalization—an explanation with which some of the mothers agreed.

Among those who retained the psychiatric-illness interpretation were some who attempted to minimize its seriousness or stigmatizing potential. Although the wife's troubles were seen as mental illness, mental illness itself was presented as something neither shameful nor unusual. George Yale mentions one occasion when "this woman said something that pleased Mary. . . . She told her that it's just like an operation, that there's nothing wrong with it, and nothing to be ashamed of." Louis Rand attempted to minimize the seriousness of his wife's hospitalization by stressing its shortness: he remarked at one point, "she got out in a short time, didn't she?" The interviewer evaded his question by commenting that it was about four weeks, wasn't it?—and Mrs. Rand said it was four weeks and two days.

Indirect attempts at minimization included the use of humor to refer to the episode:

Rands (joint): [interviewer describes her recent fall from a horse] Mr Rand asked if any damage was done beside the contusion. I said, not that I know of, but if I begin to act differently in the future I can always blame the falling off the horse. Everybody laughed here, and Mrs Rand said in a rather loud voice, chuckling all the while, "And I can always say that I've been to Napa." There was a silence after this, and then Mrs Rand changed the subject.

Finally, mental hospitalization could be minimized by the claim that the people inside the hospital were or are no worse than those outside. Wanda Karr, for example, claimed that she had never been frightened by the behavior of patients because "people outside" generally acted worse.

BLAME

Another way in which a past psychiatric history can be neutralized is by transferring the source of trouble from the former patient to others in her social circle. As I noted earlier, these women felt guilty during the hospital phase for betraying their families and blamed themselves for the troubles that beset them. But eventually some of them learned to shift the blame onto other shoulders.

The shifting of blame took two forms. First, while in the mental hospital the women learned that their psychiatric condition had an etiology, and that that etiology had to do with their family of origin. They compared notes with other women who at first felt blameworthy and learned that others shared their experiences. Second, as ex-patients their anger at inpatient psychiatric control came to be expressed against the psychiatric profession. It is also worth noting that the concept of blame is itself somewhat normalizing: blaming someone for one's troubles is also to locate them presumptively in the ordinariness and moral frameworks of everyday life.

The women learned at Napa that their troubles originated in early childhood rejection, abandonment, or mistreatment by mothers (and sometimes fathers). Joan Baker said, "My father couldn't stand me." Six months after Wanda Karr's release, Mr. Karr was blaming her mother, and her mother was blaming Mr. Karr. Similarly, Rita Vick blamed her mother: "If she had shown a little bit of love and understanding I might have been a different person." The original researchers, from their psychodynamic perspective, agreed with assessments such as Rita's (Sampson et al. 1964). The mothers themselves, however, did not. According to the researchers' records, Rita's mother "says she is tired of hearing the argument that mental illness is due to childhood and to parents—she's tired of people making trouble for themselves and then blaming others. However Rita insists that parents are responsible."

Psychodynamic interpretations of this sort, while they shift blame, remain psychiatrically grounded. The troubles in question are still psychiatric troubles; it is simply that they are caused by faulty parents rather than a faulty self. Other forms of blame shifting instead transform the grounds of trouble from the psychiatric to the everyday; in such cases, the others blamed were not mothers but husbands and psychiatrists.

Some of the Bay Area women, like Peggy Sand, blamed their husbands for their troubles prior to hospitalization: others learned to blame them during the processes of hospitalization and separation. While in the mental hospital, many of the wives felt deeply betrayed by their husbands (Goffman 1961). On release, those wives and husbands who wanted to restore their marriages had to bury a number of feelings and memories, among them the wives' anger at this betrayal. Wives who had earlier felt betrayed by their husbands in effect shifted the blame elsewhere during the ex-patient stage, in particular to their psychiatrists. Intimate relationships and feelings of resentment do not sit well together; when they coexist, blame will often by shifted. Once removed from her home to the hospital, the fifties female patient was less free to blame the psychiatrist than she was to blame her husband, since she had shifted the source of her dependence from husband to psychiatrist. As Robert Perruci indicates, mental patients are in a structurally ambivalent position vis-à-vis hospital staff: while completely dependent on them for help, they are under their domination and control:

If a patient openly rejects the idea that the staff is working for the good of the patient, then he must also accept the hopelessness of his situation. At the same time, however, it is difficult to view the staff as totally altruistic and benevolent when they are responsible for the very conditions of unfreedom that sometimes make life difficult for the patients. (1974, 54)

The analogy between mental patienthood and the fifties family is clear; the structural ambivalence of both social places fosters a sense of resentment and blame. The fifties wife was economically and emotionally dependent on her husband and dared not accept that he had anything but her best interests at heart. While close to her heart, in a sense, her husband was the most proximate source of the conditions of unfreedom that made life difficult for her. And the "therapeutic relationship" between patient and psychiatrist mirrored the position of the man and woman in the traditional family (Chesler 1972).

Under these conditions of dependence and need, resentment could safely be directed at the absent betrayer-husband during hospitalization but could not safely be directed at the psychiatrist. The reverse was true in the ex-patient stage, at least in those marriages that were continuing. Thus it is not surprising that a number of the ex-patients shifted the blame for their hospitalization to psychiatrists, to their treatments and prescriptions. Eve Low, for example, came increasingly to blame her outpatient psychiatrist (a woman): "I realize I'm putting the blame on her . . . I realize also that if I have any insight I can put a lot of blame on myself too. . . . The more I think about that woman [psychiatrist] the more of a joke I think she is."

Some of the husbands, including Mr. Low and Mr. White, enthusiastically supported the blaming of psychiatrists. Not only did it let the husbands off the hook, but it served to repair any damage to the marriage involved in blaming the woman's social situation.

Despite the psychodynamic interpretations of trouble learned in the hospital and the ex-patient's blaming psychiatrists, many women continued to blame themselves for their own schizophrenia. Shirley Arlen, for example, said that "she herself is mostly to blame for the troubles she has caused herself and her family. . . . She is different from other people, and deserving of her husband's insults and condemnation." This sort of self-blame reflects a society in which troubles are seen as individual matters and in which difficulties in gender roles and relationships are translated into personal inadequacies.

Authoritative transformation of lay persons' frames of reference by medical experts cannot be taken for granted. Such transformations take place within preexisting cultural and marital contexts of interpretation. The biographies of the individuals involved and the history of their relationships shaped their response to medicalization. We see in the responses of the Bay Area wives and husbands both action and reaction in historical context. Although in the fifties medicine was regarded as authoritative—perhaps one of the most authoritative interpretive schemes in the culture, though not as much as it is in the eighties—it was not authoritative enough to shape fully the way in which mental patients and their families came to understand their lives. Both structure in history and the process of action in response to history are important elements in understanding the dynamics of interpretation.

CHAPTER 8

The Damaged Self

In Erving Goffman's classic analysis of stigma, mental illness and mental patienthood are used to exemplify the social situation of the discredited. The labeling of mental illness, he argues, renders problematic not only a person's opportunities and interactions but also the self-image of the mental patient. In previous chapters, I have examined the ways in which the process of schizophrenic diagnosis and hospitalization affected the family relationships of the Bay Area women. In this chapter I will assess their experience of stigma—of the damaged self.

Stigma is an ungendered theory, and it is historical only by implication. But the process of stigmatization takes place within a historical context, and the participants in it are gendered. The options that are narrowed by the possession of discreditable attributes and the tension that occurs in interaction are both affected by gender—and reflexively so. For example, in eras in which married women do not work outside the home, they will not be expected, as former patients, to encounter stigma from bosses and workmates. Social circles are shaped by structural circumstances.

There are a number of social circles, with varying social distance, into which mental patients typically return following hospitalization: circles within which the anticipation and actual experience of stigma are quite variable. At the outer edge of everyday interaction are strangers and acquaintances in passing social encounters; in such situations, the discreditably stigmatized are protected by the invisibility of their label. Should this invisibility somehow be broached, however, the ex-patient may experience tension in encounters or discrimination, such as refusal of a new job or of a driver's license. Secrecy about one's past is a common response of the discreditable (Goffman 1963).

Beyond strangers, an ex-patient's social circles may be divided into those who know about the hospitalization episode and those who do not. Friends, neighbors, extended family, and those in close proximity to the prepatient's everyday life may be brought into the process of hospitalization or excluded from it; in the postpatient stage, previously unaware persons may be made aware, or become aware, of the other's changed status.

Finally, the closest social circle to the ex-patient is the family: the immediate household of husband and children and—for those families in which kin is most prominent—perhaps some members of the extended but nonhousehold family. The husband and the parents of the Bay Area women were always drawn into the hospital awareness context, whereas the children (see epilogue) and remoter kin sometimes were not.

The Bay Area women, in the posthospital phase and sometimes before, anticipated or experienced stigma in social encounters with acquaintances and strangers, in tense encounters and in restricted opportunities. Their everyday lives were, however, more profoundly affected by the private sphere of husband and children to which they returned, as housewives, after hospitalization. Within the family, kid-glove treatment—the soft stigma of intimacy—reflected back to them a sense of damaged selves as surely as did the fear or hostility of strangers. And the women experienced an internal sense of themselves as damaged, in response both to their treatment by others and to their own self-image both before hospitalization, as women, and after hospitalization, as female ex-patients.

Stigma

In his work on mental patients and others (1961), Goffman has provided us with a model of the ways in which audiences of strangers, intimates, and the "wise" respond to those who embody social damage. The typical stigmatizing reaction is that of the stranger who recoils with fear and loathing from the damaged social object (Goffman 1961; Scheff 1966). Intimates may react in various ways depending on their relationship with the person, ways that range from denial of the stigma to reinforcement of it.

The Bay Area patients were aware that "society as a whole" held ex-patients in disrepute and that their neighbors, friends, and work associates might shun or fear them. Part of their fear was based on their own pretrouble reactions to former mental patients or to the topic of mental illness in general, which were far from positive. Both during the hospital phase and afterward the Bay Area women expressed fears of stigmatization out in the community. The anticipation of such humiliation was very disturbing to the Bay Area women during their hospital stay. They were concerned both about practical matters such as the effects of hospitalization on their possible future employment, or getting a driver's license and about the feelings elicited by being feared or shunned. Furthermore, they were worried about these problems spreading to their loved ones, just as they were concerned about the psychological effects of hospitalization on their children.

Stigma in the ex-patient phase of the moral career tended to be less of a problem than they anticipated. Neither the women's life options nor their relations with people who knew their history were dramatically affected, with a few exceptions:

A neighbor and Rita Vick were watching television; the neighbor, not knowing that Rita was an ex-patient, said of the mental hospital being discussed on TV: "once you get in there you are done for." Rita then revealed herself as an ex-patient, after some fearful deliberation, and in Rita's view, the neighbor is much less friendly and even acts as if she is afraid of Rita.

The relative lack of problems in this area was connected to the fact that they were traditional housewives who spent most of their time in the home rather than in more public settings. In that sense, there was no audience of strangers to censure or shun them. Those women who did have problems with discrimination were those whose posthospital adjustment included a movement toward independence with, in some cases, attempts to sign contracts or obtain driver's licenses or jobs.

I noted in chapter 3 that the social circles of the neighborhood were prominent in some of the Bay Area women's prepatient distress. When they returned from the mental hospital, they returned not only to their families but also to their neighborhoods and networks of association. Although the neighbors (perhaps carefully and with hyperawareness) did not generally treat these ex-patients in any specially tense manner, the ex-patients themselves felt tense. Shame and embarrassment are the emotional coinage of self-stigmatization in one's public stance.

SHAME AND EMBARRASSMENT

As I noted in earlier chapters, the women's and couples' attempts to change their social circumstances—by moving house, changing social circles, or denying hospitalization—met with very limited success. As a consequence, the posthospital environment was, for these women, saturated with reminders not only of hospitalization but of what they had said and done prior to admission. Some had forgotten the details of their prepatient behavior under the influence of ECT and did not want to be reminded (though they often were). But many women experienced feelings of shame and embarrassment reflected back to them by the looking glass of self.

One element of this self-stigmatization was the guilt these women felt at having betrayed their families (and, in a few cases, at having harmed their children). As Arlie Russell Hochschild points out, guilt "upholds feeling rules from the inside; it is an internal acknowledgment of an unpaid debt" (1983, 82). Shame and embarrassment, by contrast, uphold feeling rules from the outside; they are the internal acknowledgment of a civic social debt. As ex-mental patients, relieved of moral responsibility by the sick role, the Bay Area women were officially guiltless; as discredited persons, however, they were fully open to shame and embarrassment.

As ex-patients, the women had to face the shame of both their actions and their status. As Ruth Quinn commented, "I'm so ashamed about being admitted to Napa State Hospital. It seems such a terrible thing to buck when I get out." And in looking back on her fire-setting, Donna Urey said:

"[the fireman] asked me—do you own what you set on fire? And I said, yes I do. He put me to shame right there and then. I felt awful. Of course after being questioned for awhile I started laughing—I just felt like laughing—that's why I think most of these people thought I was drunk because I felt there was a little demon inside of me or something. It was awful. I'm very ashamed of it now . . . I think it was awful shameful of me—I acted like a little two-year-old during the whole process of setting the fire."

As the emotional face of stigma, shame reveals the dependence of the stigmatized on the audience—in fact a range of dependencies. One can be dependent on the spousal audience for emotional and financial support; on employers for income; and on neighbors for civil inattention. If such is the case then women—especially housewives—would be expected to feel more ashamed than men. And those whose stigma remains secret would feel less shame than those more fully exposed.

This subject has been studied by anthropologists. Shaming as a public act of stigmatization and the attendant feelings of shame are significant modes of social control in societies in which there is a high degree of community, emotional, and material interdependence. And, as with the scarlet letter embroidered on the dress of the adulteress in Puritan America, females have generally been more the target of shaming than men and have felt more shame. The same is true of children; Donna Urey, in saying that she acted "like a little two-year-old," reflected her sense that her actions had reduced her claims to competent adulthood.

Embarrassment is the surface expression of shameful feelings, seen in social interactions and public situations. As Norman Denzin notes, our deep feelings reflect the core, inner emotions of self and morality: "Guilt, shame and resentment are deep feelings" (1983, 407). By contrast, embarrassment is a surface feeling, likely to be painful, but only momentarily so. Embarrassment was occasioned among the Bay Area ex-patients upon encountering people who might recall their prehospital behavior, which they had come to view as bizarre or delusional. Persons who caused embarrassment were avoided by the ex-patient if they could be: the Whites changed their church so Kate could avoid the minister, whom she had insisted, in the hospital phase, that she was married to. Eve Low expressed both stigma and embarrassment fears:

"I was just dreading meeting those people [relatives] after being in the hospital, and the delusions I had were embarrassing. . . . I knew that they . . . felt very badly about it and that they would try very hard to make me think that they thought nothing of it . . . they are bending over backwards to be very nice to me . . . you worry about it, what will people think, now that you've been out at Napa."

Both shame and embarrassment may be experienced vicariously, on another's behalf. Embarrassment reflects the mutual expectation of civil propriety; one can be embarrassed even for a stranger who falls flat on her face in a store. Vicarious shame, instead, is more often related to intimacy networks, where the actions of one member can cast a shadow on the moral character of another. Thus, parents typically feel ashamed of stigmatized offspring. Among the Bay Area respondents, Wanda Karr reported her mother's shame and her stepfather's hostility:

She said that her mother was "ashamed" that she had been in a state hospital. She mentioned another recent incident in which the mother was talking about someone who might need hospitalization, and Wanda said of course they could go to a state hospital. Her stepfather said to this they only have "nuts" there. She responded, "Thanks for telling me what I am."

INTIMACY, STIGMA, AND DENIAL

The type of stigmatizing hostility expressed by Wanda's stepfather may be expected in remoter social circles, but it is not anticipated among one's intimates—the "wise" (Goffman 1963). When it occurs, it is a function of the hostile person's current self-interest. It may be done to increase that person's power in a relationship, a form of one-upmanship that trades on social damage. The class of intimates said by the Bay Area respondents to respond most often in a stigmatizing manner was the mother-in-law. The women gave many examples of mother-in-law hostility: as one interviewer reported, "Rose Price complains that her mother-in-law will call her and say 'Did you have a tantrum today?' Rose will say no, and she will reply 'Well you better watch that you don't.' She also comes over 'to check'—one time she said 'I'd better stay a while, you might hurt the children.'"

The original Bay Area analysts, Harold Sampson, Robert Towne, and Sheldon Messinger, interpreted mother-in-law hostility as an expression of the traditional triadic relationship among a son, his mother, and his wife. The Bay Area respondents' family networks were characterized by various permutations of overdependence and anger: typically, the Bay Area wives were overdependent on their own mothers, while a number of their husbands were overdependent on theirs. Thus, the family stage was set both for the Bay Area patients to be subjected to their own mothers' authority—in addition to their husbands'—and for the mothers-in-law to feel hostile toward their daughters-in-law. The interviews, as well as the previous book on these schizophrenic women (Sampson et al. 1964), portray a number of families in which the primary emotional tie was between mother and son or mother and daughter, rather than between husband and wife.

Intimate stigma may be deeply embedded in the role structure of a relationship, or it may be transitory and occasioned by a particular incident or situation. The posthospital interviews include a number of occasions on which husbands lashed out in anger at their wives, calling them "crazy," "bedbugs," or some such unenlightened term for mental illness. Children, too, occasionally lashed out at their mothers' madness. Like any other condition or status, a stigmatizing one can be called into play during family conflict, often to the regret of the user once the quarrel is over. But in general, denial is a more common response than stigma in the most intimate of social circles.

As Thomas Scheff has shown for the process of mental illness, denial is the reverse of stigmatization or labeling. It involves the observation of behavior that might reasonably be labeled as crazy, followed by a denial that it indeed represents craziness (1966). Denial follows the opposite pattern in human interactions to stigmatization: while denial is less likely in encounters between strangers, it is more likely in relations among intimates. Among the Bay Area respondents, denial was the characteristic response of husbands and mothers.

Denial of mental illness, like intimate stigma, suggests a relational agenda. As indicated previously, husbands' denial of their wives' mental hospitalization or continued difficulties was related to their desire for return to the status quo ante, for separation or divorce, or for continued domestic support services. Denial on the part of the Bay Area women's mothers seemed to be related—as in the case of a few of the husbands— to feelings of guilt and shame. These feelings, in turn, reflected the special position mothers in our society are said to occupy in relation to the shaping of their children's identities.

The Bay Area patients' mothers provided a clear contrast to their mothers-in-law with respect to negative stereotyping. Instead of stigmatizing the ex-patients, most of the mothers insisted that there was nothing wrong with their offspring. In effect, they denied mental illness: Rose Price reported, " 'My mother-in-law gives me the feeling she thinks I'm crazy' . . . her mother, on the other hand, had been reassuring and told her . . . that people no longer look at things the same way." Even at the lower to middle end of the social class spectrum represented by the Bay Area respondents, these mothers were aware of the psychiatric theories that attribute mental illness to parental upbringing. Furthermore, these women knew that others would blame them for their daughters' illness:

Rita Vick: "My mother said, 'why did you let that happen to yourself? [the hospital episode]. You're not all that sick.' She says that the doctors at [the hospital] are all crazy, that it isn't true. What bothers her is that all these things that have happened and eventually my going to Napa all stems down to when I was a child."

Eve Low: "Mother says forget it now, that's all past experience, but to me, I will never forget it, I don't want to, I want to know why."

AVOIDING STIGMA

The avoidance of stigma depends on its context; thus, secrecy about the hospital episode may suffice for acquaintances, but is hardly viable within the family. Indeed, among those women who attempted to obtain employment after hospitalization three kept the episode secret; this was easier to accomplish for fifties women than for men, since women could account for gaps in their work experience on the grounds of housewifery. Similarly, women who attempted to obtain driver's licenses or sign contracts (to sell the marital home, for example) kept quiet, where possible, about their ex-patient status.

Avoiding interactional stigma was easy with strangers, more difficult where intimates were concerned. The most common way to avoid intimate stigma was to rearrange social circles to exclude or modify interaction with the offending intimates. If people close to one were the source of discomfort they became less close; at the same time, others became more so:

George Yale: (according to Mr. Yale, his wife) always felt uninclined to want to get together with people just to talk. Currently, she feels that people would be trying to analyze her. She did not feel this way with this couple whom they had known only casually. . . . who are openhearted, and open about everything. She might feel, and be right, that our close friends will studiously avoid the subject of her hospitalization entirely. He doesn't know if she feels that, or if it is true, but that is the way he thinks it would go. "I suppose if I were in their place, I probably would act like that. I don't know. It's going to be interesting to see how they act. The two times that we saw close friends on a brief visit, [husband] didn't say anything, and neither did [wife]. They told Mary she was looking fine."

The designation by intimates of mental illness as "like any other" was initially welcome in interaction with the former patients' social circles, functioning as a way to avoid the negative implications of ex-patient status. While still stigmatized by the unenlightened, the ex-patient was reassured of her essential normality by the enlightened. Over time, however, the reiteration of such reassurances began to serve the opposite function: that of reminding the ex-patient of the intimate's continued awareness of the problem. At this point the composition of social circles might once more be rearranged.

In the most intimate circles, stigma avoidance is impossible without radical reorganization of one's life. Although it is possible to change one's friends or even to move far away from one's mother-in-law, it may be impossible to avoid one's own children's taunts about craziness or one's husband's use of the hospitalization episode as a weapon in marital conflict. Although stigma and denial are opposite extremes of reaction to a particular type of behavior or attribute (Scheff 1966), the denial of stigma represents yet another means of avoiding it. If one can demonstrate that stigmatization has not occurred, then perhaps the existence of social damage can be denied. The following joint interview with the Lows, discussing a Christmastime family reunion, illustrates the theme of denying stigma within a more generalized context of denial:

Chester Low: "I don't think there was any reaction at all. *Eve Low:* "That's not possible. . . . There has to be some kind of reaction." *Chester Low:* "Well, nothing was said about it." *Eve Low:* "Nothing has to be said." *Chester Low:* "They've been very nice about it." *Eve Low:* "Aunt said to me, 'Now you be a good girl or I'll spank you.'" (Regarding the children) *Eve Low:* "I think this has been hard on them." *Chester Low:* "Yes, but . . . they very easily forget things." *Eve Low:* "That's the common conception but I don't think it is true." *Chester Low:* "Well I would say that they do." (Mr. Low wants Eve to have hypnosis to forget the hospital and its worries) *Eve Low:* "I don't think I want to forget it because I'm afraid that if I forgot it———." *Chester Low:* (interrupts) "If you forgot it and everything that led up to it you'd have no worries." *Eve Low:* "Now, that doesn't make sense."

Avoiding stigma became less of an issue as time passed. The resumption of roles and relationships in the women's social circles, the dropping away of stigmatizing encounters and people, and the distancing devices adopted by respondents served to diminish fear and discomfort as the months away from Napa multiplied. As Joan Baker commented, "I worried about what people would think when I got out of the hospital, but now I just don't care." And Rita Vick indicated that "her former concern about the stigma of mental illness has disappeared for the most part. She feels people no longer treat her differently but are quite natural with her." As we will see in the epilogue, however, time did not fully eliminate the stigma of ex-patienthood or the kid-glove treatment characteristically observed in the ex-patient's family.

Kid-Glove Treatment

While stigma is a hostile response to ex-patienthood on the part of strangers or intimates, kid-glove treatment is, on the surface, a much more benign response—a sort of stigma in disguise. The term was used by the respondents and the original interviewers to designate a soft and careful response to the former patient on the part of family members. While hostile stigma frames the individual as someone ugly as well as damaged, kid-glove treatment frames her as valuably fragile—but nonetheless still damaged.

Underlying kid-glove treatment is hyperawareness in interaction. Goffman says that the stigmatized person "may perceive, usually quite correctly, that whatever others profess, they do not really 'accept' him and are not ready to make contact with him on 'equal grounds'" (1963,

7). The others are aware of their nonacceptance, which heightens their awareness of everything concerned with the mental illness episode: Nelson White said that he was "now more aware of what he says to his wife and what she says to him. He tends to analyze things and wonders, 'is it normal, does it seem all right?'" Further, the ex-patients are aware of the others' awareness. A cycle is created that involves continual reinforcement of relatives and husbands' consciousness of the hospital episode; ex-patients' consciousness of this awareness; and husbands' and others' attempts to act as if nothing were out of the ordinary. Intimates viewed the released wives as highly fragile, but attempted to act as if they didn't; the wives were perfectly aware of their pretense:

Mrs. White's husband had continuing concern over his wife's behavior, constantly searched it for signs, and was sensitive to remarks of others that might upset her or might suggest to her that she continued to be crazy. However, he felt impelled to disguise his concern, lest the concern itself communicates to his wife that he considers her still sick or may relapse.

Donna Urey described the combination of stigma and kid-glove treatment within her social circle and the ways in which she changed her routines to avoid tension:

"Even the family now, there are times when they come over—'now what mood is she going to be in today, and what shall we do when she suddenly gets flare, or'—I mean there's always a question there and no doubt about it . . . the family . . . may not say anything you know, brings it forward to what they're thinking in the back of their minds but afterwards I get the feeling—well my husband he says 'now you made them uncomfortable and what are you going to do about it?' . . . 'you have an apology to make,' or 'you know you shouldn't have done it in the first place.' So I get it from one or the other. . . . I think (people) stop and think a lot more than they used to about my reactions to them and their reactions to me. . . . Albert still has the thought—in the back of his mind—about the fire. I'll tell you right out now. He's scared for the children's sake and he has always thought that, and I told him that as long as you have that feeling in your mind you better get rid of it . . . when we have a disagreement, that is when it is brought out to the surface (mistrust of her), other than that it usually doesn't arise . . . when we are arguing . . . (he says things like) 'well if you don't straighten out I'll take you back tomorrow and that's the end of it.' . . . He uses it over my head, and there are other times when . . . he says 'I have something over your head' but he doesn't exactly come out and say that it's that. . . . Well before they ever come over, if I know that they are coming over, which people now since I've been absent from home, have more or less called before they do arrive and let us know that they are coming so that way it gives them time to figure out what they can expect from us. . . . To know exactly what we should talk about or how comfortable we can make them feel."

In the context of the traditional fifties family, kid-glove treatment connoted not only gentleness but also the childlike and dependent status of women, a status that was exacerbated by experiences of mental illness. This was expressed both directly and indirectly. Several of the women complained that their husbands infantilized them:

Rose Price: She says that her husband treated her like a kid; he said "I told you to open the car door, now do it."

Mary Yale: "George seems to make me more nervous now than he used to. I notice it every time he gets a little bit upset, and it makes me upset too. Sometimes I can see him trying not to get upset." He treats her "like a two-year-old" since hospitalization, she says.

Just as a parent is deliberately patient and nice to a willful child, almost all the husbands "handled their wives with care" in the posthospital stage, especially immediately after release. As Mr. Mark said, "she is in the best of spirits, and I hope to keep her that way."

Husbands attempted to be tender and nice to their wives in those arenas of interaction which they saw as contributing to their wives' breakdowns in the first place. First, the husbands attempted to be more tolerant of their wives' behavior and not respond negatively to things that annoyed them prior to hospitalization. Second, they attempted to be more communicative, attentive, and responsive to their wives' emotional needs. Third, they tried to participate more in housework. Finally, they attempted to monitor their own conduct carefully in order to avoid actions that would annoy their wives. In an example of the second sort of change, Mary Yale noted that:

they have been eating out weekly recently. "That's quite a coup" she said with a laugh. Eating out has been something (husband) has not enjoyed very much, though "we do now and he does seem to enjoy it. It's something— he wants us to eat out because he feels (pause)—He does it because he wants to please me and be helpful instead of talking about money so much. He's trying not to make money such a big issue."

And despite his "plans" to divorce his wife, Mr. Quinn controlled his own behavior so as not to "upset" her:

I asked Mr. Quinn if he had discussed his plans with her and he replied, "I mentioned it once over light and I didn't dwell on it. I saw it was disturbing her and I thought that's the last thing I want to do is get her all riled up. I think I ended up saying well you get well and then we'll talk about it further. . . . It seemed to upset her but I think the weak explanation I gave her sort of salved the thing over."

These "nice" attitudes and behavior rarely lasted for the duration of the interview period. In April, for example, Mary Yale and her husband were eating out more because Mary's husband wanted to please her; she had complained about this prior to hospitalization. By June the Yales were no longer eating out. Similarly, Rita Vick said of the change in her husband since the immediate posthospital period: "I think he is losing patience or something. Instead of understanding like he used to he fires right back at me." Within the context of a highly patterned intimate relationship, it is difficult to effect permanent change.

The predominance of kid-glove treatment over hostility on the part of husbands—even those, such as Mr. Quinn, uncommitted to the marriage—tells us something about marital expectations in the fifties. It is clear from the interviews that the husbands saw kid-glove treatment as the appropriate response to their wives. Even occasional repudiation of the response was embedded in a notion of its cultural appropriateness; as Mr. Quinn said of his wife, "I talked sharply with her (on a hospital visit). I didn't try to placate her." Conversely, when the kid gloves slipped in momentary anger or distress, these husbands felt guilty and ashamed. After an argument, for example, Mr. Yale said, "I felt pretty bad that I had been emotional . . . putting so much pressure on her."

The wives' reactions to being treated with care and courtesy, awareness and paternalism, were mixed. As Goffman says, the very existence of a kid-glove treatment calls attention to the damaged self (1963). While grateful for the specific changes made in their husbands' behavior— helping with the housework or agreeing to eat out—the women were disturbed by the more pervasive implications of continuing emotional fragility. Even niceness could be burdensome. Kate White said that she felt "killed by sweetness" on the part of her husband following release. And those wives pleased by niceness resented being treated as different and handled with care:

Rose Price: "It holds quite a stigma if you have been in a mental hospital. And I don't think that's right. I don't feel like I'm a criminal because I had been mentally ill. Like [husband] and his mother and a few friends of ours that know it, if I say or do something they make me feel I am not responsible for what I do. If I say red is black they will agree with me. They are afraid they will upset me or I'll do something. I don't know what. They treat me different than they did before I went into the hospital. . . . Like we were discussing here one evening that I want to learn to drive, to go to driving school. [Husband] said no, not yet, I'm too nervous. He didn't think it was a good idea. And then my mother-in-law says, 'The first thing you know you will see something and get excited and have a wreck and kill people on the street.' So if they don't have confidence in me, how can I have any in myself?"

Although fragility treatment was sometimes resented, it appeared to have had some uses. Eve Low, whose husband had been encouraging her to go to work, found in her posthospital fragility an excuse for remaining in the home: "I think unless I change quite a bit, or until I have more insight and so on, I don't think I should go back into teaching . . . I have too many complexes." Mary Yale found that fragility treatment at work provided her with needed leeway to keep her job while experiencing stress. When asked if she felt she was treated any differently at work by her boss and his wife, who knew about her hospitalization, she said, "No, I haven't. The second day I worked [the boss] said that if I felt myself getting upset I could just tell them and take time off if I needed it. I don't feel it was condescension or anything."

MONITORING AND TESTING

The hyperawareness characteristic of ex-patienthood gave rise to a network of monitoring and testing processes within these families. Husbands not only monitored their wives' conduct, they also monitored their own responses in order to try not to be accused of kid-glove treatment. Paul Mark said of his wife, "I always try to answer her quickly so that she won't think I'm sitting there and thinking about my response." And the wives themselves monitored their own behavior and feelings for signs of getting better or worse.

As we have come to expect, the monitoring of conduct focused on the performance of household roles. The husbands watched their wives covertly, pretending not to, while the wives analyzed their own conduct and feelings. Not doing housework at all, or doing it without enthusiasm; being tired after performing routine chores, depression and crying, were all signals, for the women, of possible trouble. Eve Low noted, "I had been keeping everything [tidy] but then . . . the last week I did let everything go . . . and particularly the ironing . . . each day I noticed that I was quite tired."

The women also monitored their behavior in an anticipatory fashion, refraining from actions that might be interpreted as signs of craziness. Louis Rand recounted an incident in which "This neighbor . . . had gone in [to the garage] and taken the [gas can]. Ann had heard . . . the noise that he made. However she didn't want to say anything about it . . . as she was afraid she might be thought 'goofy.'" Desired appearances of normality were also planned. Shirley Arlen said, "If I can go home from leave and take care of two children—I mean if I can push myself that far just once—I mean I know it's going to give James confidence." As this comment indicates, the women set tests for themselves in order to prove that they were no longer crazy; and their husbands did the same. Mr. Noon said of his wife's impending home visit: "One reason I want her out is to test her. If she goes visiting with [the brother-in-law with whom she had had an affair] . . . she'll be up there a long time, she'll never get out." And Shirley Arlen described her husband's testing of her adult social competence, saying, "That's the first time I've been in a restaurant [since Napa] and my husband felt proud of me because I went."

Monitoring and testing clearly are obstacles to the restoration of a sense of normality. This was most obvious in those cases in which the process was overt. Nelson White, for example, explained how his wife "has repeated several times that the children act funny toward her." Instead of paranoia, he said, her feeling was probably "my fault" since before Kate returned home he instructed the children to "watch her" and treat her with kid gloves. Overt monitoring, testing, and self-monitoring reflected back to the woman a sense of fragility; such caution is not a feature of routine family life. While it helped restore former roles, kid-glove treatment underlined and emphasized the damaged self.

The Damaged Self

As in the image of the looking glass, the careful, hyperaware or hostile responses of others to her ex-patienthood affected the former patient's sense of self. Furthermore, this sense of self was one already eroded by women's place in the traditional social order, by economic and emotional dependence, and by the location of identity in others' actions and reactions. The damaged self of the female ex-patient was a consequence not only of mental illness and hospitalization but also of the more general situation of women in fifties America.

As indicated earlier, Goffman distinguishes between the discredited visible stigma of race or handicap—of status—and the discreditable invisible stigma of ex-patienthood or homosexuality (1963). Setting his theory within a specific historical context, I have argued that gender, like "tribal" affiliations and "abominations of the body," was a basis for interaction problems and the limitation of opportunities in the fifties; indeed, it remains so today (Schur 1984). Women in the fifties were legally and economically disadvantaged in a number of ways, most particularly in receiving approximately forty cents for every dollar men earned (Margolis 1984). And women were also victims of that form of stigmatizing interaction, sometimes reserved for children, servants, and old people, which Goffman designates "nonperson treatment" (1963).

For the Bay Area women, the stigma of ex-patienthood represented one episode in the complex biographical progression of gender, age, social class, and other forms of disadvantage. It is not surprising, therefore, that their inner experience of a damaged self, and its outer expression, were not limited to their moral career as a mental patient. Damage permeated their lives from childhood on.

This is not to say that all the women felt damaged prior to the experience of being labeled mentally ill. Rather, the fifties provided a context in which damage to the female self was a likely outcome, and in which a "traditional" rhetoric obscured its structural sources. In the absence of a feminist ideology that could give legitimate expression to their distress, the women expressed a sense of disjunction from the social order, of being "out of place," strange, or alien in the world—as, indeed, in the prevailing social order, they were. Shirley Arlen said, "Sometimes I feel happy but it seems like I'm still looking for something, to make it complete—my husband's got money, a good job, my kids are healthy, and I mean—my husband will give me anything I want—I can't see what it is that I want." This fundamental sense of dislocation was a source of worry to these women and prompted a search for some culturally idiomatic explanation:

Joyce Noon: "Maybe . . . I never did grow up or something. Maybe something is wrong with me. I don't like it. . . . Mel does such a good job,

and—everything—but it's me you know. 'cause I'm just like I am. . . .
If he had somebody just like him he might be happy too. I don't know. All
he wants is me. Maybe I—I don't know—maybe I didn't grow up or
something."

For these women the traditional female role was a place that they occupied, but it was not really their own.

Edwin Schur points out that the sick role itself is identified with
women and that this identification renders women weak: "The very
expectation that females will perpetually have ailments reinforces wom-
en's lack of self-confidence and self-sufficiency" (1984, 243). More specifically, the mentally ill role is associated with females; this too has
generalized consequences for the place of women in the social order:

women have had to confront the stigma . . . of perpetual exposure to being
labeled mentally ill. To an extent, this stigma indirectly affects all women.
The general tendency to treat women as being emotionally disturbed is
always present in the background as a ground for dismissing what a woman
says or does, and as an implicit "threat" should she seriously step out of line.
. . . If women embrace their assigned role fully they are regarded as overdependent, narcissistic and neurotic; if they reject it, they are seen as schizophrenic. (ibid., 199)

Being hospitalized exacerbated these women's sense of strangeness in
the world and gave it a name and shape. As Dorothy Smith says of the
psychiatric interpretation of women's trouble, "Resentment and despair
are not treated as valid responses to her situation. The realities of her
situation as she feels them are not treated as valid" (1978, 7). The
schizophrenic label and hospitalization amplified the Bay Area women's
sense of abasement and lack of entitlement in comparison to their
husbands. Mary Yale described the typical course of marital conflict in
the Yale household:

"When something comes up in the house about (child) or anything we don't
agree on it's not a very pleasant situation. It turns into a personality thing.
Not constructive; it doesn't get anyplace. Usually (husband) reacts by

telling me I criticize everything he says and everything he does. I don't think so, but he evidently feels so." She contemplated her own prehospital tendency to get on a "kick" of criticizing him, and her lack of entitlement to do so in the light of hospitalization: "I'll probably get on a kick now and start criticizing him all over the place." She paused. I remained silent. "Somehow I don't feel that I have any right to criticize now—I haven't been functioning myself for so long."

Although Napa provided a moratorium from their roles for these women, it validated anew their sense of worthlessness and not belonging:

Shirley Arlen: "Sometimes I think I'm going to be in here the rest of my life. I don't know how to change—I don't know what to do with myself. I want not to be lazy. I want to do things. I want to know if I did push myself—and if I did feel tired, and still I had something to do—if I did I would feel better instead of laying down—I would do it—I'm afraid to take any chances now, I'm so scared, I'm afraid to do anything. I don't know what to do . . . I'm afraid of raising my children . . . I'm afraid that I'll hurt them—that I'll raise them to be mental patients too. . . . I don't want them to grow up like me."

Cora Thorne expressed the same sense of worthlessness and fear for her child, locating it in the dependencies of gender. She attempted to kill herself and her daughter, she said, because of her unhappiness about her husband's desertion and her desire that her daughter would not grow up to be a woman "hurt" the way she had been by men.

In the social context of the fifties, repair to the damaged self of the female ex-patient was possible only in the most limited arena. Unable to change social structures and gender roles—indeed only dimly aware of their constraints—the women attempted to change their social circumstances and their selves. As Shirley Arlen said when asked what she expected or wanted from hospitalization: "to be a new woman when I walk out of here." When pressed further on what ways she would like to be a new woman she responded, "in every way, I guess." Some of the husbands echoed the wish for a "new woman" as their wife; more commonly, however, the "old self" of the competent housewife was what they wanted. Paul Mark said, "She is as normal as can be—acts just like she used to before she started getting sick. . . . She starts a job like [making] a dress, she finishes it now, instead of throwing it away. . . . And she don't cry any more like she used to."

Although psychiatric hospitalization in the fifties reinforced the lessons of familial dependence, it also undermined them, in part through psychiatry's very focus on self-analysis. And although the self-reliant patient was a latent theme within the medical model, the self-reliant wife did not fit within the confines of the traditional family. Wives were expected to subordinate their needs and wants to those of their husbands and children; a wife and mother was expected not to be self-absorbed and selfish. This expectation conflicted with the idea that to become and stay well the ex-patient had to do a lot of thinking and analyzing, and exert self-will and self-control. It also conflicted with the ideas of independent action that had been learned as part of therapy. Both the women and their husbands spoke in the ex-patient phase of problems in the readjustment of dependency patterns: while most of the spouses welcomed a return to the traditional balance, some did not. In a joint interview, "Mr Price said, 'I'm responsible for you' . . . this touched off an explosion. . . . 'I'll be taking care of you next time—nobody is responsible for me' said Mrs Price. A huge squabble followed all this." But for most—wives and husbands alike—their troubles came to be seen as caused by the wife's selfishness and desires for independence; thus the remedy was not the self-absorption of therapy and "thinking" but a reabsorption of the woman's self into her role:

Joan Baker: "I think I have just let myself get in such a rut, thinking no one loved me or wanted me, because I didn't get any attention. I wanted my husband to notice me and take me places, which he never did."

Eve Low: "I feel like baking cookies and things that take more . . . trouble and time and that's because I've made up my mind to be a homemaker instead of always worrying about a career."

Ultimately, all the Bay Area women were either restored, like Eve Low, to the traditional housewife role, or left, like Joan Baker and Ruth Quinn (and later Donna Urey, as will be seen in the epilogue), without a viable social place. And despite the wishes of these women and their husbands, neither the self nor the marital relationship was fundamentally changed by the hospital experience, since both were embedded in the structure of the fifties family. These women's selves were most clearly damaged not by hospitalization but by gender and by their place in those most intimate social circles that could—under other sociohistorical conditions—have provided succor. The social situation of families in capitalist-state societies is such that with intimacy comes not only a sense of order, a place for the self (Berger and Kellner 1970), but also stress and alienation. This was particularly the case for fifties women, since their situation was both obdurate economically and legitimated ideologically. Today, although women are still housewives, they do possess more economic independence than thirty years ago, and they can draw on the ideology of feminism to understand the sources of the damaged female self.

Thus, coming full circle, we see that the damaged self is a process embedded not only in one's family life but in the temper of the times. Both men and women were damaged in the fifties, but women more so. And while all women were affected to one degree or another, the sharpest experience of distress occurred among those women who suffered other blows in addition to gender. Poverty and social class took their toll on women; schizophrenia and mental hospitalization took theirs. The damaged self, in the final analysis, is the product of history, of the social order, and of the flawed way of being within which we come to experience our most intimate understanding of ourselves, our lovers, and our children.

Thirteen Years After

What became of the schizophrenic women and their families as the traditional ways of the 1950s were challenged by the political radicalism of the 1960s, and the resurgence of feminism in the 1970s? Although we have only glimpses of their lives after Napa from the 1972 reinterviews, these glimpses are worth recording for what they tell us about biography and history. The changes in these women's lives—and in the lives of their husbands and children—reflected changes in the social structure: in the place of women within marriage, the home, and the workplace; in psychiatry and mental-health policies; in feminist legitimation of women's protest against their traditional place. The continuities in their lives, and the flow of one generation into another, tell us something about the reproduction of social problems over time.

The Women

Between the 1950s and the 1970s, the lives of the Bay Area women changed as all lives changed; but these changes were patterned to some degree by the earlier crisis. Furthermore, there were fundamental changes in the place of women at work outside the home between the fifties and the seventies, though the place of the housewife changed less (see chapter 1). By 1972 at least eight of the Bay Area women were working or had worked outside the home. Two of the divorced women—

Kate White and Mary Yale—had careers. The still-married women worked to "keep busy" or "earn a little extra" in pink- or blue-collar occupations: Shirley Arlen and Louise Oren as cashiers or bookkeepers, Rita Vick and Joyce Noon (before her 1969 death) as waitresses ("off and on"), Peggy Sand as a cocktail waitress in her husband's restaurant, and Ann Rand (before her suicide in 1971) as an assistant in her husband's furniture shop.

Traditional objections to women's work persisted in some of the marriages, with the wife's history of mental illness used as an additional rationale for her not working. Joyce Noon commented in the 1972 reinterview that she had been offered a job in a doughnut shop recently, "but her husband told her not to take it. In addition, she was worried that work would be too much for her: 'I wanted to, but I'm leery. . . . Don't think that I'm that far along yet . . . it might throw me back.'" Although Mr. Arlen had "allowed" his wife to work for the past sixteen months "he seemed to resent her working, saying that 'she doesn't have time to do her housework and I have to make dinner for the boys.'"

What had not changed over the years was that these women were still housewives. Whether they worked outside the home or not, all the women said that they were responsible for the basic household chores of childrearing (in those families that still had children at home) and housework. Wanda Karr, for example, said that she did all the household tasks and that her husband "never helps. Once in a while he cooks. Sometimes, if someone is coming, he picks up." When she was sick, "he didn't do anything then . . . he wouldn't even pay the bills, even after the second and third notice." Furthermore, the inequality, boredom, and isolation of the housewife role continued to precipitate emotional stress among some of the women. Mr. James traced Irene's most recent crisis, in March 1972, to his taking a moonlighting job from two to ten in the evening, at which time Irene was left "alone and isolated"; Irene herself complained of always "hanging around the house."

Several of the couples were divorced or separated by 1972: the Whites, the Yales, the Vicks, and the Ureys. Other couples, such as the Sands, remained married despite decades of serious difficulties. Indeed, the 1972 interviewers' assessment of some of the enduring Bay Area marriages was that they were fundamentally unchanged since the earlier study, characterized either by symbiotic dependence or equally symbiotic hostility:

Both the Sands said they had nothing in common, neither interests nor activities. . . . The idea of change in her marriage frightened Mrs Sand: "I'm not sure that after this long time if he really changed it would do me any good because when you live with a certain thing so long it's hard to let go." . . . Both spouses agreed that they were still as sexually incompatible as they were fifteen years ago, and that there was nothing to be done about it. Mrs Sand remained isolated from all but family contacts because "He made it too uncomfortable for me to have friends of my own or any activities outside of those that pertained to him."

Though the Sands were an exception, the "separate-worlds" marital adaptation of the fifties seemed to have changed, for some of the couples, into some form of eternal togetherness. Among the eleven couples whom the researchers had classified as "separate," at least four were, in 1972, inhabiting the same one: the Noons, Rands, Thornes, and Karrs. In three of these families this new symbiosis was precipitated by the husband's retirement from work, perhaps indicating that social structure—the separation of home and workplace—was responsible for the separate-worlds adaptation. The fusion theme of these dyads was expressed by several of the spouses:

Joyce Noon said that her husband likes bowling, but "if I can't do it, he can't do it." She used to fear he would leave her but he has invested so much in making the marriage work that she no longer has that fear.

Mrs Rand's previous pattern of dependency on her husband had continued throughout the 1960s. She was with him both at home and at work, and either avoided other people altogether or socialized with them only if he was also there. . . . He had retired from his upholstery business . . . prior to the interview . . . partly because he wanted to be able to devote all his time to his wife. At the time of retirement they bought a house "to find a new pattern of life" and to be closer to relatives, and because Mrs Rand's doctor thought the move would be good for her.

Besides the eleven separate-worlds marriages, the original researchers had characterized four of the relationships—the Yales, the Karrs, the Lows and the Arlens—as symbiotically triadic, merged trigenerational marriages. In these marriages, the parent of one of the spouses literally came between husband and wife, arrogating many of the wife's role functions (Sampson et al. 1964, 37–40). Over the years, elderly parents had died or moved away, and young children had become adults; thus, the alliances and symbioses in these marriages had changed. Sometimes, merged families became symbiotic dyads, as in the case of the Karrs. But in most of the families, the generational dynamics had moved toward greater intimacy with adult offspring rather than husbands. Shirley Arlen, for example, said that she was "close to no one. Only my children." And Peggy Sand had formed an alliance with one of her daughters against her husband, who in turn allied himself with the other daughter.

Some of the Bay Area women were no longer traditional housewives at the time of the reinterview: Kate White, Mary Yale, Rita Vick, and Donna Urey. Kate White and Mary Yale both embarked on careers as photographers after their divorces. Kate White commented that "being successful at my work" was her greatest pleasure in life. Mary Yale said that she liked her work because it was challenging and enabled her to "contribute . . . express my own ideas." While the lives of both these women had obviously changed considerably since their original hospitalization, only Kate White identified to any degree with the newly emerging feminist movement. She said that she would not be interested in remarriage because "she felt that most men exploit women, and after all her therapy, and her involvement in a career and in 'women's lib' she could not tolerate exploitation by a man."

Rita Vick and Donna Urey had very different experiences with divorce and independence. At the time of the reinterview, Rita Vick was unemployed and living on 318 dollars per month welfare, supplemented by

Medi-Cal and some housekeeping service from the welfare department. She had worked as a waitress off and on in 1962 and 1963 but had found it difficult to work "because I can't stick to anything." Although Donna Urey could not be contacted for a reinterview, her husband said that she had entered a board-and-care home after their divorce, and had subsequently remarried at least three times. Although independence may be positive for some women who feel trapped in traditional roles, other women released from their husbands' control—and particularly ex-patients—may find themselves without the necessities of life.

THE MENTAL HEALTH SYSTEM

Changes in the mental-health system also provided the context for changes in these women's experiences with psychiatric treatment. Regulations concerning informed consent to treatment altered the ratio of voluntary to involuntary treatment in California's state mental hospitals and—at least in theory—made patients more knowledgeable about their treatment. The quicker release of patients from the state mental hospitals, coupled with the attempt to maintain them on psychoactive drugs, rendered hospitalization a decreasingly viable means for the Bay Area couples to cope with their personal and marital problems. Indeed, Mr. Noon complained about the stringency of commitment procedures in 1972 as compared with 1958. He had found it increasingly difficult to commit Joyce to Napa as a solution to their marital conflicts, though he sometimes succeeded: according to the 1972 data, "His strategy . . . was to make her mad and keep her mad so that 'the doctor will see how unreasonable she is' and allow him to commit her. He lamented the changes in mental health law, saying that he used to put her in Napa when she got 'difficult,' but 'now they won't let me put her in Napa, it's almost impossible.'" Over the years, both Noons had used Napa as a resource in their marital battles. On Mrs. Noon's third hospitalization, in 1959, the admission notes read: "Husband threatens to return her to hospital if she doesn't agree with him. Patient shows no signs of acute distress upon return. . . . Problem seen by doctor as marital." A 1969 admission note read: "returned home by the county. Not sick. Husband is ill." For her part, Mrs. Noon said that she went to the mental hospital when she "can't cope; it is an asylum, a place where no one bothers you and you get away from your problems."

Most of the Bay Area women had been rehospitalized by 1972, though with decreasing frequency over time (see appendix A). Joyce Noon had the most total hospitalizations—eleven—while Peggy Sand and Wanda Karr had no rehospitalizations. A number of the women had had outpatient individual or group psychotherapy or been maintained on psychoactive drugs; only Donna Urey had any experience with the growing system of board-and-care homes for the chronically mentally ill. Although outpatient therapy still posed problems financially (insurance coverage continued to favor inpatient treatment even in the seventies), the community mental-health center movement did provide more services than the fifties equivalents. Most of the women had had some sort of outpatient therapy, either individual, group (including some self-help), or marital over the years since their first admission to Napa; several reported that they valued self-help or group therapy for its sociable aspect. As in the fifties, a couple of the husbands had become threatened by their wives' individual therapy. Mr. Arlen had, according to Mrs. Arlen, attended one of her therapy sessions, and "hated" the guy; he did not understand her relationship with the therapist and didn't like her discussing her problem with an "outsider." He "made" her stop seeing him.

Medication seemed to have lived up to its ameliorative claims for some of these women. Interestingly enough, Kate White—who had been uncertain whether she was crazy or just ambitious in the fifties—regarded herself, in 1972, as having been "psychotic" and as still in need of medication. She took stelazine and artane daily, saying that the drugs helped her because, without them, "I feel things too deeply . . . tense and unable to cope." In addition, a number of the husbands appreciated the impact of psychoactive drugs on their wives' role performance and general state of mind. Mr. Thorne said that his wife "definitely" functioned better when she was on stelazine than when she was not, while Mr. Noon complained that toward the end of her two-week prolyxin shots his wife "doesn't want to do anything" by way of housework. Mr. James saw his wife as currently improved as a result of the pills she was taking, among which he named librium, elavil, hormone pills, thyroid, and tofranil. Indeed, in contrast to the fifties, the respondents—and especially the husbands—seemed to be able to name and evaluate the drugs they took, which reflects the new era of informed consent to treatment.

Another change that has occurred in the state mental hospital system since the fifties is the almost complete cessation of ECT use. (Although ECT is used very rarely in California's state mental hospitals, its use has increased in California's private hospitals since at least the mid-seventies [Warren 1987a].) There are no recorded instances of the respondents receiving ECT after the sixties (see appendix A). Although a few of the women who received ECT saw it as having helped them (Shirley Arlen, for example), for most it remained one of the most painful and threatening of hospital memories. In 1972 Wanda Karr said:

"I remember the clamps on my head, the sparks as it started, and I was very frightened. Afterwards I woke up with the most terrible headache I ever had. It was like being hit on the head with a bat. It was really an awful experience." . . . She said that immediately after the last shock she couldn't remember things, but she doesn't know about the others since she doesn't remember the treatments at all. In talking about memory she said, "you know I can't remember anything about the hospital" or the birth of her daughter.

For this patient, at least, long-term memory was affected by ECT, thirteen years after.

LOOKING BACK

When asked to reflect back on the Napa experience and its impact on their lives, and on what precipitated their troubles—the moral career of the mental patient—the women gave diverse accounts. A number of them, from the vantage point of the seventies, recognized woman's traditional place as the source of stress. In looking back at the troubles that precipitated her hospitalization, Mrs. Arlen referred to "not wanting to live—pregnancy and undesirable marriage—I was upset, nervous and miserable even after hospitalization and had to struggle to get well." Kate White said that she had had "a personality conflict—a desire to write, to have a career, to work, as well as a home life. . . . I felt trapped, and then panic at the trapped, bored feeling. At the hospital I could feel safe from the pressures . . . [she had] deeply missed work, and couldn't adjust to the role of supportive wife of a businessman."

The respondents attributed positive changes in themselves and in their marriages to the Napa episode. Joyce Noon said that her marriage had become stronger because of her hospitalization; the family "all pulled together" to help her get well and thus had grown closer. She had changed, too, from the experience; she said that prior to her first hospitalization she did not know her husband or pay attention to him as she did now. But she also indicated that she had "lost part of her life—youth" because of hospitalization. Finally, some of the women denied that hospitalization had had any effect on themselves or their lives, or only a minor impact. Peggy Sand contrasted Napa's impact on her with its impact on her marriage:

"I really don't think I've changed at all, although it may have been at that point I started to become a little more aggressive, not so reserved . . . [hospitalization] just gave him something else to pound me with . . . perhaps being removed from the situation was helpful. . . . He always said if I did what I should we wouldn't have any trouble . . . at first he felt I didn't belong there [Napa] at all, he wanted me to come home, when it suited his purpose he signed me in there, to keep me under his thumb."

Mrs. Sand added that if she could do it all over again differently she would have filed for divorce, but that this would only have been possible if she had been raised differently.

Despite the passage of time, stigma was still a problem for the Bay

Area women, especially if they had had several hospitalizations. Some kept their ex-patient status secret from new social circles, while others did not or remained within those circles who knew about it anyway. Kate White, in moving from California back to her home state, left her psychiatric history behind her. She avoided the stigma of ex-patienthood in her career by not admitting to it, although she said that her current employer probably knew about it. Interestingly, she kept the episode secret from even very close new friends, on the grounds that knowing about her status would change the way they treated her and the way she behaved:

It is important to keep the secret because "people in such a situation tend to overcompensate in order to prove to people that they're well now. That feeling creates a fake kind of personality." Her problems are generally attributed by others to her divorce and the patient allows this rather than reveal her hospitalization. She wants to avoid feeling "apologetic" which she did earlier [in California, before her move].

Those women who could not or would not move into new social circles faced the problems of having their histories known so well analyzed by Goffman in *Stigma* (1963). Shirley Arlen said that she had had some trouble obtaining a driver's license when a background check revealed her history; Ann Rand had had the same problem when she applied for a civil-service job. Interestingly, even the tenor of interaction was still affected by ex-patienthood thirteen years later; Shirley Arlen said that although her mental hospitalization had made "no difference" to her friends, her family was still "uncomfortable" and perhaps ashamed. Wanda Karr said that her friends and neighbors had caused her no difficulties, with the exception of one church acquaintance who "treated me like I was from outer space." Mr. Noon said that his wife's hospitalization had made a difference to some of the people they knew: "yes it has—some have turned away. The ones that come around treat her like anyone else."

Kid-glove treatment persisted over time in several families. Mr.

James said that his wife did not discuss the hospitalization episode because "it disturbs her. She does bring it up once in a while for a few minutes, but I do not initiate any discussion of it." Joyce Noon said that her husband "keeps things that would worry her to himself" and that she had had a problem with him treating her "like a child" and telling her exactly what to do. Mr. Karr monitored his own behavior toward his wife for signs that he was treating her with kid gloves and thus reflected fragility back to her. A researcher reported, "They discuss everything. If he were to avoid certain topics like her hospitalization she would become angry at being treated like she was at all different or had to be handled in a special manner." And yet the ex-patients did reflect back their sense of being handled by people in a special manner; even if that special manner was one of niceness, or helpfulness, it was also the echo of stigma. For example, "Shirley Arlen's neighbors are 'nice' [about the hospitalization]. . . . her family treats her differently, not a 'natural atmosphere.'" Similarly, Joyce Noon said of her neighbors' attitude to her hospitalization, "They don't think it's nothing because I've always been acting all right. . . . Anyone who knows has always tried to be helpful."

The Husbands

The husbands of the Bay Area women have been absent from these pages as subjects; they have been heard only as commentators on their wives. But it is clear that the male role in the traditional fifties family, as well as the female, was often ambivalently experienced. All the Bay Area men worried, in the fifties, about not having enough money to support their families; their cultural manhood depended on their wives' not working, and yet their economic circumstances begged for additional resources. Being a housewife was a source of stress for women in the fifties; having to earn a living and support a family was a source of stress for men. Some of the men, like some of the women, dreamed from time to time of role reversal—of escape, of staying home. Mr. White wanted to take a year to write a novel and take care of the children while his wife worked. Mr. Yale said wistfully, during his wife's original hospitalization: "I'm supposed to be the head of the family—the one that does, and makes the decisions, and sometimes I want her to make them. Sometimes I want her to do things I'm supposed to do."

Looking back at their lives and marriages from the perspective of the seventies, many of the Bay Area husbands exhibited a degree of tenacity and commitment in their marriages in the face of adversity, something that is becoming increasingly rare in contemporary life (Bellah et al. 1985). Some of these husbands seemed to have functioned as guardians to their wives over the years, both in the sense of control and in the sense of care. One of the husbands wanted to protect his wife even from the reinterview; distancing the mental hospital was still important to this couple's adaptation:

Mrs Thorne was not reinterviewed, and Mr Thorne's interview was a telephone one, obtained only with difficulty. He stated that they had been through "one of those" before and he wanted no part of it. He said they were trying to forget all that. When I asked whether he would at least be willing to give me a little information over the phone, he asked me for information about myself and how I had gotten access to them.

The husbands almost uniformly complained of the toll their wives' psychiatric disabilities had taken on their role performance: their work. Mr. Noon, for example, attributed his recent demotion from driver to fare collector in the bus company to worry about his wife, which made him fall asleep at the wheel. But he also said, "I wanted to fight the whole world to get her well. Didn't marry her to get a divorce." He claimed that he did not want Joyce to work not because he feared her independence but for her sake: "She wanted to work but he 'talks her out of it, she's not able . . . she would fail and then be humiliated.'"

Only Mr. Karr and Mr. Sand said that their wives' hospitalization had not had any impact on their lives or role performance as workers, and only Mr. Urey rated the impact of his ex-wife's hospitalization as "very positive." Before her hospitalization he had been an auto mechanic, which he hated. The welfare aid that Mrs. Urey obtained after her first hospitalization had enabled him to go to school and eventually to get a job as an auto salesman. In 1972, he was teaching auto shop in high school.

Those husbands who had divorced or in some other way repudiated their wives seemed only in part to bear the guilt of the traditional fifties husband; by 1972, the ideology and social legitimacy of divorce had changed. Although neither Rose Price nor her husband could be reached for an interview, records indicate that Rose remained at Napa from July 1959 until January 1964 because no relative, including her husband, would take her home even though the hospital wanted to discharge her. Both Mr. White and Mr. Urey, in describing the divorce process, used the rhetoric of therapy and self-realization to justify their action rather than the pre-sixties language of commitment and tenacity (see Bellah et al. 1985), though Mr. Urey also said that he had felt "guilty as hell" for abandoning Donna and getting involved with another woman. He commented:

I was pretty selfish. . . . I felt that I just couldn't go through that anymore myself, having to worry about her . . . the kids, trying to work. . . . Sometimes when I would come home the house would be in shambles. . . . Sometimes she would, out of the blue, throw something through the window. . . . The voices, that came back after she came back, but I could deal with that pretty well. But there was always the fear in me that it would get back to what it did originally . . . [when] she set fire to the house."

While there was commitment and tenacity in some of these marriages, there was also violence. Mary Yale, who had once again in 1972 recently separated from her husband, said that he could not tolerate her having friends and treated her like a child. He criticized her for spending money and for "being fat," and threatened her with violence when she attempted to contact a lawyer about divorce. Mr. Yale admitted to hitting his wife but claimed that it was her fault because she was "a master of sarcasm and had a biting tongue." And Mrs. Sand said that her husband used to beat her and their two daughters but had controlled his violence over the past few years.

In some of the families, blame for the women's troubles had been relocated in their husbands' overuse of alcohol. Mr. Sand and Mr. Oren had continued to drink heavily for several years following the original study. While Mr. Sand had "cut down on his drinking" in recent years, according to his wife (and despite working as a bartender), Mr. Oren had not. Indeed, Mrs. Oren attributed their marital difficulties and her four hospitalization episodes to his drinking. She said that "her current sensation of wanting to die [was] related to her husband's drinking. She felt depressed and troubled whenever his drinking 'gets bad' . . . when asked by the interviewer if she had attempted to communicate with her husband about this she replied 'No, he'd just say it [mental illness] was happening to me again.'"

Aside from Mr. Urey and Mr. White, the men did not seek assistance for their emotional troubles; the only exception was for drinking and—if pressed by their wives—marital therapy. Mr. Oren had been to Alcoholics Anonymous "off and on" for years, while Mrs. Oren had recently joined Al Anon (which she enjoyed both for therapy and for sociability). Although his drinking was not seen as a problem for the Ureys in the fifties, Mr. Urey reported in 1972 that he had been a member of Alcoholics Anonymous for some years and was currently an abstinent alcoholic. Two of the couples attempted marital therapy in the years after Napa. These attempts were as short-lived as they had been in the fifties. The Sands had tried marital therapy in the sixties, but Mr. Sand had refused to continue, so Peggy continued in individual counseling. Mr. Sand explained his lack of involvement as a lack of belief in therapy, saying, "Problems must be settled by those involved. No outsider can really know what's going on in other people's lives . . . this leads to more trouble . . . [my wife] feels differently . . . that talking to a counselor or even a friend helps."

Although many of these marriages were troubled, going to marital therapy was not an option for most of the couples, either because they were not part of the therapeutic culture or because the men disliked therapeutic—as well as marital—forms of intimate communication. For two of the husbands, however, the psychiatrization of everyday life had amplified over the decade. Mr. Urey had been in psychoanalysis for the past three years in addition to his membership in Alcoholics Anonymous. He had been in "lots of groups" of the self-help variety and referred to his recent shoulder pains as a "conversion symptom" to "cop out" of dealing emotionally with his financial troubles. In 1972 Mr. White was training to be a psychotherapist. Life experiences with psychiatry had, for these men, intersected with the growth of a therapeutic culture in America (Bellah et al. 1985).

LOOKING BACK

The husbands, like the wives, were asked to assess retrospectively what they saw as the cause of the women's schizophrenia and the impact of hospitalization. Interestingly, a number of the husbands in 1972 located their wives' earlier troubles in the stress and demands of the traditional housewife role. Mr. Urey said, "as I look back on it now, I think much of it was that she never had time to recuperate from one child to the next. . . . Getting married young . . . early in our life she had an affair with my brother and a couple of others." Mr. Yale said of Mary that "she never got her freedom" and simply transferred her "dependence from her father to her husband." Mr. Arlen said that his wife had had an "identity crisis. Too young to accept the responsibilities of wife and mother." He added that she "has grown up a lot, is able to perform her responsibilities and role functions adequately." Other husbands attributed their wives' troubles to the sorts of contingencies discussed earlier, from menopause to the annoying behavior of neighbors.

To some of those husbands who had remained married, like Mr. James, their wives seemed "the same—no different" as a result of hospitalization, while to still others the women, or the marriages were "better than ever." And, as had been the case thirteen years earlier, at least one husband professed himself uninterested in the whole matter, not noticing anything: "Mr Arlen said that he did not remember what led up to his wife's rehospitalization and did not know how she felt. He did say that his wife interpreted her own stress as a product of marital conflict; he felt, however, that his wife tended to blow up situations out of proportion."

A couple of the husbands said that their feelings for their wives changed because hospitalization had made the women "different." In discussing his divorce, Mr. Yale said that his feelings for Mary changed after hospitalization because "'she had changed—she was not the same person . . . the burden of her problems threw a shadow over my feelings for her so that it sort of took over.' ECT was, according to Mr Yale, responsible for these changes; after ECT Mary "seemed to care only about conforming . . . it was a loss of a tremendous person, very talented . . . afterwards, nothing." Mr. Urey made a similar analysis of his divorce:

He said that when they got married his wife was a very happy, motherly and non-violent person, but that "the experiences in the hospital . . . I feel like they sapped the strength out of her . . . I think they were giving her shock . . . I saw her one week and she seemed in good spirits, and the next week she was a complete vegetable. When she came home there was still that characteristic—a whole kind of doped up, very passive, very tranquil, spaced out place."

Mr. Urey and several of the other husbands also referred to the bitterness they had felt—and the damaging effect on their marriages—when mental hospitalization did not effect a cure: "where I really got bitter was the second time, when she went into [county hospital] and I felt, 'well, you copped out again' in my mind. . . . I assumed she would go there [the first admission, to Napa] and come back and everything would be great. And that never happened." Mr. James agreed with Mrs.

James that their hopes for the future had been dashed by her relapse after the initial hospitalization, and were disappointed in its lack of effect.

A continuing theme in the fifties and the 1972 interviews alike was, for both husbands and wives, their assertion that Napa provided them no information about the woman's condition. Neither the patients nor their husbands had been able to converse freely with the ever-busy doctors, and staff members claimed they were unable to provide information without a physician's approval. Mr. Urey was one who remained bitter about this aspect of the hospitalization episode. The Napa psychiatrists, he said, "really turned me off," asking, in response to his requests for their medical opinions, "well, what do *you* think?"

The Children

There were both changes and continuities in the lives of the Bay Area families from the fifties to the seventies—in work and leisure, sex and money, psychiatric treatment and patterns of marital communication. One additional area of change for all the couples was their children's growing up, a process that inevitably had an impact on their dyadic patterns. Mr. Sand's comments on his marriage and on his children exemplify both changes and continuities in general, and the specific impact of children on marital patterns:

He described his wife as "lazy," just like the younger daughter; their older daughter he referred to as "full of energy and initiative, just like me." . . . He said that he and his wife were in conflict over everything, with him getting angry and her withdrawing, then both getting "revengeful." This pattern, he said, has remained unchanged over the years. He wished that his wife would "express herself, stop running away, and do more housework" and that she would like him to stop talking to women in the restaurant.

Neither wish, he added, was likely to be granted. . . . Both Mr and Mrs Sand agreed that Mrs Sand and their youngest daughter had "banded together" in a conflictful coalition against Mr Sand.

The children of the Bay Area study are even more shadowy than the husbands, since they were rarely interviewed. There are simply glimpses of them in the original interviews as they pestered their parents or played with the interviewer's tape recorder. But both in the fifties and in the seventies the parents spoke about their children and the ways the Napa experience affected them. In both cases, the crucial factors seemed to be the age of the child at the time of the first admission and the adequacy of the caretaking that was arranged for him or her during and after hospitalization. And throughout the thirteen years of their children's growing up, the mothers bore the guilt of what they feared was faulty mothering.

The families in the fifties sometimes told their children about the mental hospitalization and sometimes did not; the older the child, the more likely he or she was to be informed. Younger children were regarded as more adaptable and less apt to be worried about finding out something that had been kept secret. Joan Baker, for example, said that her seven-year-old was unaffected by her hospitalization but that her twelve-year-old daughter would not come and see her at Napa because "she's afraid I might be like those people . . . and [that] I might die." Later in 1958 she added that her oldest daughter "cries all the time because I'm here" and had tried to commit suicide by swallowing aspirin. Some of these older children were quite nasty to their mothers about the episode. Eve Low said that "her eldest sneers about her house and personal sloppiness before hospitalization, and being in a robe at noon. Eve told her she should be more understanding." And Mrs. Baker, whose eldest daughter was "unhappy and difficult," reported that she had said to her, 'Why don't you go back to Napa?' . . . Anything that goes wrong I am [to my daughter] either a Napa nut or a filthy liar or a beer guzzler."

But the main problem for these women in the fifties—the one that followed them over the decades—was the long-term impact of hospitalization on their children's lives. In the 1972 follow-up the respondents were asked to comment on the outcome of these fears: the perceived impact of hospitalization on the next generation.

In our culture, schizophrenia and mental hospitalization are seen as damaging over the generations, either genetically or behaviorally. Thus, the women who were divorced had trouble over the custody of their children, since their husbands were in a position to make an issue of their psychiatric history. Although in the sixties and seventies women were still overwhelmingly awarded custody of their offspring, two of the Bay Area women—Donna Urey and Rita Vick—lost theirs to their husbands. Mrs. Vick, however, successfully renewed the custody battle for her fourteen- and fifteen-year-old sons a year later. She commented that the boys were frightened of her for at least a year after that because their father had told them that she was "crazy" and would hurt them. Mrs. Vick had not seen her twelve-year-old daughter since her husband "took off" with her when she was eighteen months old.

For the Bay Area respondents, only the process of time and maturation could provide reassurance that their children were all right despite their mothers' troubles. The mothers' psychiatric history represented a readily available explanation for those troubles that their children had as they grew into adolescence and adulthood. Mrs. Vick expressed her surprise that—in view of her violence and psychiatric history—her two boys were "all right." Mr. Urey, by contrast, said that his elder daughter (then twenty-two) resented him because he imposed a mother role on her during Donna's hospitalization. He described one of their twin sons as "schizophrenic" and the other as "in therapy." But he minimized the impact of his wife's hospitalization on the children, blaming his twenty-year-old twin son's schizophrenia on his recent contact with her: "he is the only one I think it had an impact on, being in contact with his mother. I think that most of the kids have blocked out anything that they saw previously."

Most of the families attributed some of the problems their children had growing up to the earlier crisis. Mrs. Sand said that her elder daughter was obese because her father "is one of her problems and one of mine too." The elder daughter had complained that Mrs. Sand wasn't available to her while she was growing up. Mrs. Sand agreed:

I wasn't available because I was reading or in such a depressed state of mind that I had no time for [the children's] problems. The fact that I did drive to Napa on her birthday, she's never . . . or maybe she has gotten over it. . . . [At the time of hospitalization] the children must have been confused in addition to a host of other emotions—at the time, I didn't have anything left for them.

As in the fifties, the respondents believed that the effect of hospitalization on the children varied with the children's age. Mr. Karr, for example, said that he was "not concerned" about the impact of Wanda's hospitalization on their children since they had been "too young" for it to have mattered much. He added that their now fourteen- and sixteen-year-old daughters had "no problems," despite the fact that they had learned about what had happened. Mrs. Baker said that her children had been affected differently by her hospitalization, with most of the impact felt by her elder daughter—the same comment she had made thirteen years earlier.

Sometimes the children were seen as essentially normal, but were estranged from their mothers as a result of earlier events. Mr. Thorne said that the two eldest of their four children had rejected their mother and her control as a result of Mrs. Thorne's mental illness. Mrs. Noon, who had been hospitalized in the aftermath of an illicit affair with her brother-in-law, said that her son blamed her for the earlier crisis, because he still remembered her relationship with this man (he had walked in on them while they were making love). Her son, in 1972, was highly critical of her for her "smoking and sloppy housework," while her daughter-in-law was afraid to leave their infant son with Mrs. Noon because of her psychiatric history.

Because they were the ones hospitalized, and perhaps also because they were women, the Bay Area mothers were more worried about their children than the fathers were. Mr. Arlen, for example, said that the impact of hospitalization on their children (who were fourteen and fifteen in 1972) was "minimal"; Mrs. Arlen, however, commented that the children had reacted "too little" to the events and that "They are not as happy and secure as other kids." Although at the time these mothers' guilt at betraying their children had been somewhat mitigated by the adoption of the sick role, over the years guilt could be—and was—triggered again and again by any difficulties their children had while growing up. They needed continual reassurance that they had not damaged their children irrevocably:

Mr Noon said that over the years Mrs Noon had been concerned that their son would "get it"; their social worker had tried to convince her that mental illness wasn't contagious. She was finally convinced that he was "OK" and felt relieved by this.

Kate White used to worry about her children feeling unable to depend on her, "but we have gotten over that." She also used to worry that they would come to fear mental illness in themselves, so a few years ago she explained to them that her mental illness was "circumstantial," which was what her psychiatrist had told her. Although Mr White agreed that their children had no special problems, he claimed that during her many hospitalizations she failed to care for the children, who "took more care of her than she did of them."

Only an apparently "normal" progression from childhood into adulthood could ally these particular kinds of guilt and fear.

The 1972 reinterviews demonstrate a number of ways in which history repeated itself in these families, both within and across the generations. Most of the Bay Area women were still economically dependent, still housewives, and still—with the partial exception of their adult offspring—emotionally as well as spatially isolated. The marriages that persisted had changed not at all, or only in limited ways. Not only did the early schizophrenic episode have considerable impact on family life over the years, but the women were still emotionally troubled.

People who commit themselves or are committed to mental hospitals are part of (even if detached from) family structures that include earlier and later generations. And, in turn, these family structures are embedded in a historical context that shapes the psychodynamics and social roles in both the nuclear family and the family of origin. In the fifties what was significant about families was their gender-role structure: thus, gender was one of the several crucial features through which madness was experienced and by which madness was socially identified and treated as such. The Bay Area women became defined as mentally ill and in need of hospitalization within the traditional fifties family; thus the family and gender context shaped the moral career of the mental patient. In turn, mental patienthood had a profound effect on the internal dynamics of the family, though not on its essential structure. And it is these internal dynamics, together with the historical moments of the sixties and seventies, that shaped the children of the madwives.

APPENDIX A

Case Histories

Shirley Arlen

Shirley Arlen, who was twenty-six at the time of hospitalization, came from a poor urban family in which she was the fifth of eight children. Her father was "passive and dependent" and her mother "energetic . . . but a very casual housekeeper" who did little role training with Shirley. After she quit school Shirley held several unskilled jobs, all of which she left or lost after a short period of time.

Shirley and her husband James (twenty-four) had been married two years when she was hospitalized, and they had two infant sons. The marriage took place when Shirley was pregnant, possibly by another man. From the beginning of the marriage Shirley felt overwhelmed by the responsibilities and tasks it entailed: she had had no prior training in grocery shopping and handling money, and could not manage these tasks or routine housework. She felt that James, her husband, was critical of her and that she was unentitled to the use of his money since he had earned it.

The Arlens moved in with James's parents prior to the birth of their first child, and Shirley's mother-in-law took over child-rearing tasks once he was born. When Shirley became pregnant again, they decided to move into their own home. There, James took over the household chores, while Shirley stayed in bed much of the time. James took the elder child to his parents' house daily, while the younger child was cared for in the Arlens' home by Shirley's mother. Eventually the younger child and Shirley moved into her mother's home, while James went to his mother's. A week later, Shirley was hospitalized.

Shirley left the hospital after thirty-six weeks (and ECT) with renewed optimism. In the final interview thirteen months after release she was performing her household roles in a new home to the satisfaction of herself and her husband, and she felt satisfied and optmistic about life.

Shirley Arlen was rehospitalized once, for one week, in 1961 or 1962. She had also had short courses of thorazine on an outpatient basis. The Arlens were still married at the time of the 1972 reinterview, and Shirley was working as a cashier.

Joan Baker

When she was hospitalized Joan Baker was thirty-five and her husband Arnold forty-one. They had two daughters and had been married for fifteen years. Joan was a World War II "war bride" from England. Shortly after Joan had joined Arnold in the United States, he had an affair with another woman. This event, together with the combat death of one of her brothers, precipitated physical illness as well as depression.

Joan Baker had been chronically depressed about two years prior to hospitalization, feeling unloved by her husband and troubled by obesity; these problems had been exacerbated by her husband's elder brother coming to live with them. She would often visit the grounds of Napa State Hospital and watch the patients, half wanting to become one of them.

The crisis of hospitalization was precipitated by Arnold's meeting another woman at a party and going home with her. The next day the Bakers fought violently, and Arnold threatened to go and live with the other woman. Joan persuaded a friend, her husband, and the family physician to hospitalize her.

On a home visit about a month after hospitalization Joan Baker slashed her wrists superficially; upon her return to Napa she received ECT. Though in the throes of separation, the Bakers told Napa they were reconciled, and Joan was placed on indefinite leave of absence in the custody of her husband. In fact she was living alone. From a follow-up interview two years after release it appeared that Mrs. Baker was doing well, working and taking care of one daughter (the other was with her husband) and planning to be married. The Bakers were subsequently divorced.

There were no records of readmission for Mrs. Baker. She attributed her earlier hospitalization to her husband's rejection of her, which reactivated her despair at her father's earlier rejection of her. Arnold was contacted but refused to be reinterviewed.

Irene James

Irene James was forty when she was hospitalized, and her husband was forty-six. It was Irene's second and Ralph's first marriage. At the time of the first hospitalization they had been married for nine years and had a seven-year-old daughter.

Irene graduated from high school and worked until her first marriage. She had a daughter by her first husband and gave custody of the child to her mother when she got a divorce. She married Ralph when she was thirty and gave birth to her second daughter two years later; both childbirth and child rearing apparently posed considerable difficulties for her.

The crisis of hospitalization began when Irene fainted, attributing this to the "change of life" and to previous "plots" by neighbors against her. She was released from Napa after fifteen weeks, but soon "relapsed into a very withdrawn and autistic state with rambling paranoid delusions" (Sampson et al. 1964, 137). By the end of the study period she had been rehospitalized twice.

Napa and other hospital records indicate that Irene James was re-hospitalized at least four more times between 1960 and 1971. She received ECT treatments during her later hospitalizations. Neither of the Jameses could be contacted for a reinterview.

Wanda Karr

Wanda Karr was twenty-nine and her husband Richard twenty-eight when she was hospitalized. They had been married for three years and had two daughters. Mrs. Karr was described by the Bay Area inter-viewers as an "intellectually limited" woman whose elder brother was "an emotionally disturbed mental defective" (Sampson et al. 1964, 138).

The Karrs lived next door to Wanda's mother (then divorced from her father), who assumed responsibility for the Karr's household and for the elder daughter. Wanda's crisis took place upon her return home from the birth of her younger daughter, when she attempted to breast-feed and care for her herself and was not successful. At the time Wanda's mother had moved in with her, and Richard had moved next door with Wanda's stepfather.

Wanda was hospitalized for eight weeks and received ECT. On her return home the Karrs bought a house far from Wanda's mother but moved back again after a few months. At the time of the original study's follow-up interview, the interviewer commented that matters were much the same as prior to the first hospitalization, with perhaps some marginal improvement.

The Karrs were still married in 1972, and both were interviewed. Wanda had had no further hospitalizations since the original study and had not had any forms of outpatient treatment. The Karrs no longer lived close to Wanda's mother.

Eve Low

At the time of Eve's hospitalization the Lows were both thirty-eight and had been married twelve years. They had girls of ten and two and a seven-year-old boy. Eve became an elementary-school teacher because her mother wanted her to and worked briefly at teaching. She became engaged to her husband Chester the day she met him, and they were married within a month.

Eve's mother often lived with the couple and took care of house and children; Eve sometimes had to work to support the household since Chester had a history of sporadic unemployment. After the birth of their third child, Eve sought outpatient psychiatric treatment to deal with her emotional and marital problems. Her hospitalization was precipitated by her psychiatrist's leaving town and transferring her to someone else. "At this point Eve became acutely psychotic. One symptom was violent repudiation of her mother" (Sampson et al. 1964, 141).

Mrs. Low was hospitalized for eleven weeks and received three ECT treatments, which resulted in four fractured vertebrae. At the final interview twenty-one months after her release, both Eve and her husband seemed to be doing well. She was free of symptoms, while he was, for the first time, not only steadily employed but doing well in his job. Eve's mother was no longer living with them. There were no 1972 reinterviews.

June Mark

June Mark was thirty-three and her husband Paul thirty-four at the time of her hospitalization, and they had been married twelve years. It was her second marriage and his first. They had three daughters aged eleven, eight, and four. June's mother had died when she was a child.

June's first husband was from a wealthy family, while Paul was—like June herself—from a poor background. At first their marriage was close, but later it became one of separate worlds, with June absorbed in her children and Paul in his outside work and leisure activities. Paul complained continually about her spending too much money on their children.

Prior to her hospitalization June had become preoccupied with a "conspiracy" involving her children and the wealthy members of a club to which the family belonged. She developed the delusion that these club members had been "spreading rumors" that she was unfaithful to Paul and sexually promiscuous.

June Mark was hospitalized for twelve weeks and received ECT. About a month after release she resumed outpatient psychiatric treatment, receiving first drug therapy and later outpatient ECT. When interviewed two years after release Mrs. Mark was "delusional and . . . intermittently psychotic" (Sampson et al. 1964, 143) and no longer performed household or child-rearing tasks.

June Mark was rehospitalized at Napa five times between 1962 and 1966. She died of a heart attack in June 1969. Her husband was reinterviewed in 1972, and he said that they had remained married until her death, even though he had given up on having a wife and family more than fifteen years ago.

Joyce Noon

Joyce Noon was twenty-six and her husband Mel thirty-seven at the time of their marriage. They had been living together off and on for eight years, but had been married only two; their son was seven years old. Joyce's parents had been divorced when she was a child, and she spent much of her childhood in an orphanage and with various relatives. Mr. Noon had been married twice before and had a history of psychiatric treatment and one mental hospitalization. Joyce married another man and divorced him during one of the Noons' intermittent separations. In addition, Joyce was involved in an off-and-on affair with her sister's husband.

The event that led up to the crisis of hospitalization was an accident involving the Noons' son, which resulted in brain damage. Joyce began to hear voices accusing her of being a whore and sought outpatient psychiatric treatment prior to her admission to Napa. She was hospitalized for seven weeks on her first admission and rehospitalized six times during the period of the original study, receiving ECT on several of her readmissions. A hospital note for 1961 comments that her husband had written to the doctor and said that he wanted a divorce because his wife was mentally ill and had affairs. The doctor cautioned the husband to "look at the good aspects of the relationship."

Joyce Noon was rehospitalized at Napa voluntarily three more times, once in 1962 and twice in 1971. In 1972 the Noons were still married, and both Noons were reinterviewed.

On her tenth admission, in 1971, Joyce was reported as claiming that her husband was having an affair with his daughter-in-law and attributed her relapse to her son's marriage which she "could not handle." Since the last readmission she had been receiving injections of thorazine and Mellaril every two weeks, which she said "make me fall asleep all the time."

Louise Oren

When Louise Oren was admitted to Napa she was thirty and her husband Jack was thirty-two. They had been married for nine years and had two children: the son was illegitimate but he had been adopted by Jack, while the younger daughter was three. Louise's father died when she was eighteen; a year later she gave birth to her first illegitimate child, who was eleven at the time of her hospitalization.

Louise met Jack when she was pregnant with her second illegitimate

child, who was born and given up for adoption. The Orens married
secretly at that time under different names, and then remarried publicly
under their own names a year later.

The crisis of hospitalization revolved around Louise's difficulties with
sexuality and motherhood (Sampson et al. 1964). She had a brief admission to a general hospital three years before her admission to Napa,
diagnosed as in an "anxiety state"; she had cried out that her abdomen
was swelling and it would burst and she would die. The Napa hospitalization was precipitated by her attempting to choke her youngest
child.

Mrs. Oren was hospitalized for nine weeks, and was pregnant at the
final interview (she had a daughter). The interviewers commented that
"in view of her history, it may be that special trouble lies ahead"
(Sampson et al. 1964).

The Orens were still married at the time of the 1972 reinterview, and
both spouses were interviewed. Mrs. Oren had been rehospitalized once
at Napa in 1965, an event that she said was precipitated by her husband's
drinking and her feeling that she was having a heart attack. The Orens
currently had four children, the youngest daughter now four years old.
Mr. Oren said that he had never considered separation but she probably
had, especially when he had been "really drinking," which he defined as
"a pint of liquor a day."

Rose Price

Rose Price was thirty-four and her husband William forty-six at the
time of hospitalization. They had been married fourteen years, and their
three sons were aged thirteen, eleven, and four. According to her husband, Rose was fine until her first pregnancy but then began having
"spells" in which she neglected to do housework and child care. Mr.
Price assumed the role of caretaker both of his children and of his wife,

and "a pattern of chronic autism" developed in Mrs. Price (Sampson et al. 1964, 148). Just prior to hospitalization Mrs. Price became preoccupied with fears of harm coming to her youngest son and had the delusion that she was pregnant.

Mrs. Price was hospitalized for eight weeks and readmitted twice during the study period. By the end of the study, she was once more in the hospital, and her husband and children had moved to another state. Hospital records indicate that Mrs. Price remained at Napa from 1959 to 1964 despite the hospital's wish to discharge her because neither her husband nor other relative would take her in; she was finally discharged in 1966. In 1960, records indicated that she "screamed for ECT" but that the treatment was discontinued after a month because she suffered vertebral fractures. Neither Price could be located for the 1972 reinterview.

Ruth Quinn

Ruth Quinn was thirty-eight and her husband Tim thirty-six when she was hospitalized. They had been married for fourteen years and had a thirteen-year-old son and eleven-year-old daughter. Ruth's father died when she was sixteen. Ruth entered teacher training after high school, when she met Tim. After they were married and during her second pregnancy, she "felt guilty, rejected and very dependent," while Tim felt "trapped and furious toward her . . . saddled with responsibilities and blocked in his vocational and financial ambitions" (Sampson et al. 1964, 149). Ruth began to drink heavily, became fat, and neglected the housework, making at least three suicide attempts prior to hospitalization.

After she joined Alcoholics Anonymous Ruth discontinued drinking, but she continued to struggle with her weight. Prior to hospitalization Ruth's weight dropped to less than one hundred pounds and she became confused, withdrawn, and paranoid, claiming that strange things were happening. After vitamin shots failed to make her feel better, Tim lured her into Napa under the pretense of having a physical examination.

Ruth was hospitalized for five months and received ECT. The Quinns separated, and Ruth went to live with her elder sister. Twenty months after release Ruth was living alone without working or having custody of her children.

There were no records of rehospitalizations for Ruth Quinn, and neither of the Quinns could be contacted for a reinterview.

Ann Rand

When Ann Rand was hospitalized she was thirty-six and her husband Louis was thirty-seven. They had been married for thirteen years; her second marriage and his first. They had eleven- and six-year-old sons, plus Ann's sixteen-year-old son by her first marriage. Ann's parents were divorced when she was a child.

About two years prior to hospitalization Ann became restless in her housewife role and began taking junior-college courses. She became very busy, stressed, and complained of gastrointestinal troubles and insomnia. At the time of admission she was in a panic and convinced that she would die if she moved her bowels.

Ann was released after six weeks' hospitalization. After release, the Rands saw their marriage as improved, with Louis being more attentive, "helping out" with the housework, and expecting less of his wife. Mrs. Rand had applied for a civil-service job but had not yet heard the results of her test.

Records indicate that Ann Rand killed herself with her husband's shotgun in 1970. She had had no readmissions to Napa until 1970, when she had two short stays. The 1972 interview with her husband indicates that "everything was fine" until about 1969, and that he did not know what went wrong. He also said that she had attempted suicide two other times, taking pills with "a quart of whisky." She had failed to obtain the civil-service job, presumably because of her Napa record, and had continued to "help out" her husband in his furniture shop until her death.

Peggy Sand

Peggy Sand was twenty-nine and her husband Floyd thirty-six when she was hospitalized; they had been married for twelve years and had daughters aged eleven and six. As the original researchers comment (and I would not argue with the assessment), "The marriage was sadomasochistic." Peggy had thought of going to a mental hospital to escape Floyd for about three years prior to actually doing so; her admission was preceded by a particularly violent quarrel. During hospitalization, Peggy had an affair with a male patient, an event that persuaded her husband to have her committed involuntarily immediately after her release.

Peggy was at Napa for about nineteen weeks. The original researchers comment, "Sixteen months later . . . Mrs Sand was still married and living at home . . . so far as we could determine neither she nor the marriage had changed from the pathological prehospital patterns" (Sampson et al. 1964, 155).

The patterns were essentially unchanged in 1972, when both the Sands—still married to each other—were reinterviewed. As Mr. Sand said, when asked how things had been going since the last contact in 1961, "the same . . . the problems between us will always be the same. I think one way, she thinks another. Can't really ever get together." Mrs. Sand had received no further psychiatric treatment or hospitalization.

Cora Thorne

Cora and Peter Thorne were both thirty-one when she was hospitalized, and they had been married for nine years. They had a seven-year-old daughter, a five-year-old son, and an eleven-month-old one. From the time of her first pregnancy Cora had become increasingly anxious and intolerant of sexual relations; Peter had withdrawn into a separate world of involvement with work and male friends. Peter began to go out with another woman during Cora's fourth pregnancy, and his request for a divorce precipitated the crisis of hospitalization. She tried to kill herself and her daughter.

Cora miscarried, and Peter proceeded with plans for divorce, while Cora was hospitalized for twenty-nine weeks and received ECT. After some months of living alone and working, with Peter taking care of the children, Mrs. Thorne and her husband were reconciled.

The Thornes were still married at the time of the 1972 reinterview; Mr. Thorne spoke with the researcher on the phone but refused to let him talk to Cora. Records indicate that Mrs. Thorne was rehospitalized three times in 1966 for very short periods: her husband indicated that these admissions were caused by further miscarriages.

Donna Urey

Donna Urey was twenty-six and her husband Albert twenty-seven when she was hospitalized; they had been married eight years and had five children. Donna was illegitimate, and her mother abandoned her when she was eight, from which time she was raised in an orphanage.

Donna and Albert met while they were in high school and Donna was in his family as a foster child. At first their marriage was very happy, but Donna became increasingly troubled with the birth of each child. She heard voices off and on for years before she precipitated hospitalization by setting fire to her house and breaking all her dishes.

Donna had the longest hospitalization of any of the women: sixty-four weeks. She received ECT and was rehospitalized a year and a half after release, at which time she was pregnant with the Ureys' sixth child.

At the time of the 1972 survey the Ureys were divorced and Mr. Urey had custody of their six children, aged between fourteen and twenty-two: Mrs. Urey could not be reached, but Mr. Urey agreed to a reinterview. Records indicate that Mrs. Urey was rehospitalized twice at Napa in 1967, saying on her last admission that she came because "I had no place to stay." Her ex-husband said that she had gone into a board-and-care home but that she had subsequently remarried at least three times since their 1962 divorce. Mr. Urey had become involved with his present wife during Donna's second hospitalization.

Rita Vick

Rita Vick was twenty-nine and her husband Leo thirty-six at the time of her hospitalization. They had been married for three years and living together for six. Rita had been married twice previously and had had six children by four men; she had lost custody of all of them. Leo had been married once before. The Vicks had two sons, aged two and one. Rita herself was an illegitimate child and had a history of neglect and delinquency.

Rita and Leo met in a bar and began to live together within the week. After the Vicks were married Rita attempted to regain custody of one of her sons, who was in a foster home; the court gave temporary custody to the father, who took him to another state. After this event Rita was briefly admitted to the county psychiatric hospital.

Three years later Rita was admitted to Napa following the birth of her two Vick children and continuing custody battles over other children.

After final custody of one son was awarded to his father, Rita began to threaten social workers, call the police, and claim she was going crazy. She was admitted to Napa after about two weeks.

Rita remained at Napa for thirteen weeks, when she failed to return from a home visit (though she voluntarily returned after a few months). She received ECT. After Rita's final discharge the Vicks moved several times, and Rita became pregnant again. Following the birth of their third child, a daughter, Leo filed for divorce and custody of the children, claiming that his wife had beat the one-month-old baby and thrown her against the wall. About two years after release Rita was "living alone but was involved in an obscure relationship with a policewoman friend and an untrained 'psychologist' who were helping her with her problems by hypnotism" (Sampson et al. 1964, 162).

Records indicate that Rita Vick was not subsequently rehospitalized. Although Mr. Vick could not be contacted, Rita was reinterviewed in 1972. Her summary of the fifteen years between initial hospitalization and Napa was, "it's been hell!" She said that her husband had divorced her and gained custody of their three children, although she had regained custody of their two sons. She had not seen her daughter since she was eighteen months old. She added that her husband did contribute to their support, in addition to her welfare payments.

Kate White

Kate White was thirty-six and her husband Nelson thirty-eight at the time of hospitalization. They had been married for twelve years and had two daughters, aged five and two. When she married Nelson she continued her work as a reporter until the family moved abroad temporarily because of his job. On their return to the United States Kate became a housewife and mother, while Nelson (who was a professional-level, well-educated man) continued to dabble in one career after another. She began to suspect her husband of homosexuality and had an affair with another man (see Messinger and Warren 1984). The crisis itself "began shortly after the Whites bought their first home and experienced a sense that, after more than a decade of marriage, they were really settling down" (Sampson et al. 1964, 163). The symptoms that precipitated hospitalization included delusions about the homosexuality of her husband, her neighbors, and herself (Messinger and Warren 1984).

Kate was hospitalized for twenty-nine weeks and resisted return to her husband and family. When she did return to her husband, the Whites vowed to "try to settle down and 'really live like a married couple for the first time'" (Sampson et al. 1964, 164). Mrs. White, however, had several more extramarital affairs and was rehospitalized eighteen months after release. At the two-year follow-up interview, the Whites agreed that their marriage was disintegrating, and Mr. White was having an affair with his secretary.

Kate White was rehospitalized a total of nine times at Napa and Camarillo between 1957 and 1963; all but the first commitment were voluntary admissions. One 1961 admission note read, "She is very intelligent, has tried to suppress ambitions and professional drive, and in the interest of her husband and children she has found it extremely difficult to be just a housewife. Has tried to work out a plan with husband to combine professional experience with her domestic duties."

In the 1978 reinterview, Kate said that she was "in and out" of the mental hospital prior to her divorce about 1965, because of "feelings of conflict in the marriage . . . panic at the trapped, bored feeling. At the hospital I could feel safe from the pressures, from my husband's and his family's demands for the wife-mother role." In 1972, Kate White was working as a photographer and was on a maintenance dose of psychoactive drugs. Mr. White had married his secretary.

Mary Yale

Mary Yale was twenty-nine when she was hospitalized, and her husband George was thirty-four. They had been married for five years and had a four-year-old daughter. Prior to her marriage, Mary had worked as a newspaper reporter. Mary and George married after a short courtship; subsequently, George lost his job and the couple moved in with Mary's mother, though they subsequently moved to an apartment next door. Torn between her mother and her husband, Mary developed homosexual delusions and believed she was turning into a man. She sat and cried for hours. After a brief attempt at outpatient psychotherapy, she was committed to Napa.

Mary was hospitalized for eighteen weeks and received ECT. The Yales separated a few months after Mary's release, but were subsequently reconciled. Two years after her release the couple was still married, and Mary was working as a waitress.

By 1972 the Yales were again separated; both were willing to be reinterviewed. Mary had not been readmitted to Napa after a single readmission in 1959; she was working as a "photographer for a black community newspaper."

On the Intensive
Interview

The methods of the original study—the research plan, sampling procedures, data collection, and analysis—are detailed in Sampson et al. (1964); unfortunately, space limitations prohibit their elaboration here. As I indicated in the introduction, my method of analysis was that of the descriptive social scientist: documentary interpretation. What I want to add here is a few comments on what I learned during this work about the intensive interview—and in particular repeated intensive interviews—as a method of social research.

What I find most interesting about the Bay Area data are the ways they demonstrate how meaning is situated in context—both the context of the interview (as the ethnomethodologists claim) and the context of the respondent's place in the social structure (as the positivistic focus on "variables" implies). The repeated-interview design of the Bay Area research was useful in developing my understanding of the ways both structure and situation shape response. I discuss these ways in the contexts of the stages of the moral career and of the clinical meanings of research interviewing for both the individual respondent and the dyad. I then contrast this more situated view of the interview process with what I call the myth of rapport.

Interviewing in the Patient
and Ex-Patient Phases

The progress of an interview was clearly influenced by the moral career during which it took place. Most of the women welcomed their Bay Area interviewer, during the first weeks of hospitalization, as someone who was willing to spend some time with them, listen to their accounts of circumstances, and not rush in and out. Mary Yale, in her first interview, told the interviewer that "I'll jot things down to tell you. It breaks the monotony." The interviewers were valuable as visitors during the women's Napa stays because of the boredom of the hospital, with little to do, the infrequency of visitors from the outside, and the rarity of talking with someone who would not dismiss one's communications as delusions. In addition, the respondents attempted to press the researchers into service in their search for therapeutic status, since they lacked formal sources of information. The researchers attempted to avoid this role.

Ruth Quinn: At this point Mrs. Quinn said that she wants to find out how many shock treatments she has had. I asked why, and she said, "I don't remember wanting to know how many I have had—but a patient asked me. Then they discussed how many they had and somebody said she was more disturbed than the other one was." Mrs. Quinn explained that the more disturbed you are the more shock treatments you get and therefore you can judge the seriousness of somebody's condition by the number of shock treatments they have received. She has doubts that this is true, but nevertheless she is curious to know how many she has had. She asked me for my opinion and I told her I didn't think it was necessarily true that the more shock you had the more serious your condition was.

Thus, the structure of the hospital experience promoted the interest of the researcher in obtaining cooperation, though some of the emotional aspects of feeling troubled tempered this cooperation.

In the posthospital phase, the home setting more generally elicited an unwillingness to be interviewed, especially in those marital relationships in which there was an attempt to return to the relationship before trouble developed. All the interviewers commented on the way the initial at-home interview with the ex-patients changed what had become "typical" hospital interaction:

[*First joint interview with the Noons after discharge*]: I said "Hello, how are you?" Joyce reacted to this initially as an inquiry about her psychiatric condition. . . . I think she was momentarily uncertain whether the situation defined her as patient or hostess. This ambiguity, in various manifestations, plagued the three of us from time to time through the evening.

[*First ex-patient interview*]: I was trying to be informal, Mr. Oren was clearly waiting for the question–answer period to begin. . . . I felt somewhat uncomfortable in this setting and often had difficulty thinking of appropriate questions to ask.

Those respondents who wanted to forget the hospital experience displayed various degrees and kinds of resistance to the interview. By contrast, those who viewed the hospital as a place of refuge associated the interviewer with that refuge and displayed an interest in continuing the interview process. Other patients were ambivalent about the interviewer, responding on the basis of situations and moods. The most extreme case of refusal, on the part of both Lows, consisted of complete withdrawal from the interviewing process immediately after the wife was released from the hospital. In the interviewer's first telephone conversation with Mrs. Low, she insisted that the interviews would be too much of a reminder: "Eve Low said she should forget the past, continuing to see me would serve as a constant reminder of the past, and even if we did not talk about the past I would still remind her of it anyway, just by my presence." The interviewer stressed that she would not talk about the hospital or the past if Eve did not wish to, but Eve was well aware that the interviewer's presence would call up the past in her mind in any case and would thus cast discredit on the posthospital self she was endeavoring to construct. As Rose Price said, "I need people to stay out of my troubles for a while—get the house fixed up—do my own plans." And Mary Yale commented, "it makes me uncomfortable . . . you write down everything I say." Ann Rand said of the posthospital interviews that "anything is preferable to this . . . you keep asking a lot of questions. Things I want to forget about."

Several of the patients mentioned, often repeatedly over time, that the interviewer reminded them of their stigma, protesting the interview process on that basis:

June Mark tells me that she cannot fully participate in the research simply because the research in itself signifies the stigma of deviance which she is struggling to avoid. . . . "I don't like being a guinea pig . . . you keep asking a lot of questions . . . things I want to forget about. . . . It's not normal, my talking to you. . . . It's just that I'm reminded I'm a patient. If you're a patient, you're always a patient."

Indeed, there was evidence that others interpreted the continued presence of the interviewer as a sign of the former patient's continued troubles. Joan Baker commented that her daughter said to her, "You are still a Napa nut or that guy [the interviewer] wouldn't be coming here talking to you."

Many of the husbands expressed an equal dislike of the ex-patient interviews. Kate White's husband, more than a year after release, said, "I'm getting a little more reluctant to talk about it. I don't know if it's just that I'm more reluctant to talk about things, or that there's nothing to talk about." Similarly, Mr. Yale said to the interviewer, "I'd rather not talk about anything that happened seven months ago. And Mary feels the same about it. We're done with it." The interviewer asked, "Do I remind you of it?" "You do when you ask questions like that. . . . Yes. Often. I'd rather not talk about it. It's done. We both feel that way."

There were several strategies adopted by ex-patients and their husbands for expressing objections to the presence or questions of the interviewer: being difficult, verbal protest, defining the situation as social, and role reversal. Being difficult was a shifting and multifaceted strategy, hard for the interviewer to confront directly. One interviewer noted, "The Karrs have a strong desire to break contact, communicated by silence, sullenness, arranging for the continued presence of children, quiet refusal on Wanda's part to be seen separately, comments on note-taking, aggressive refusal to answer questions, queries as to the consequences of missing appointments."

Some interviewees, over time, attempted to redefine the posthospital interviews as social rather than research occasions:

Ann Rand repeated that she would only see the interviewer again if she would have her over to her house. While the interviewer was evasive, Ann said "then I suppose you still see me as a patient. To me you are either a friend or some kind of authority, now which is it? The way I see it, you either see me as a friend or a patient."

Mr. Oren asked me if I wanted to join them for dinner, and was rather insistent about this despite my repeated declining. He later invited me to drop over to his place some afternoon, bring along a broad and just let my hair down and enjoy myself. . . . I was emphasizing the fact that this was my job, probably in the hope of getting him to accept the situation as such and not redefine it.

From time to time, patients and their spouses attempted role reversal, either in a joking and tentative, or in a more determined manner. In role reversal, the interviewee took control of the situation by asking questions of the interviewer, introducing topics, or offering psychological interpretations of the interviewer:

Ann Rand (at beginning of interview): "What have you been doing?" (both laugh). As we sat down Ann said something to me like "Well, what's been happening?"

Donna Urey (to interviewer): "You look slimmer and trimmer—you've let your fingernails grow out, haven't you?"

Jack Oren said, "I think that you're a kid that missed happiness somewhere along the line." He then started speculating about my past life and thought that something had happened to me, maybe in high school, to make me feel like that. Mr. Oren first was critical about my interviewing technique, and then started to question me about my life, and so on.

In contrast to the majority of former patients and spouses, who viewed the interviewer as an occasional or persistent intrusion into the process of self-redefinition, a few patients who felt fragile continued to welcome the interviews as a form of contact with the hospital. The ways these patients communicated their desire for continued contact roughly paralleled the ways the majority discouraged contact. Instead of "being difficult"—forgetting appointments, talking in a busy room, or not talking at all—these patients were enthusiastic, talking freely or over-estimating the amount of future research contact. One interviewer recorded that "Irene James anticipated the next interview in one week, then corrected it to two weeks." Instead of role reversal or casting the researcher in the role of social caller, the patients who still felt mentally ill attempted to cast the researcher in the role of therapist or adviser. These interviewees did not want to terminate the interview process: Shirley Arlen said to her interviewer at their final meeting, "Goodbye, savior."

Interviewer: I had the feeling that Irene James was desperately trying to gain some control over her feelings and thoughts by talking about them to me, but unfortunately I did not feel that she was very successful in the attempt. Irene says that when I arrive for my interview that seems reassuring.

Interviewer: I asked Shirley Arlen if she would see a psychiatrist and she said no, she couldn't afford it, then "all she would do is talk, and she feels she would do better just talking to me."

Clinical and Research Interviewing

Although the Bay Area interviews were designed as research rather than clinical interviews, it is clear from the preceding comments that they took on a number of clinical functions for the respondents. In addition to reports by the patients that they "felt better" after talking to the Bay Area interviewers, the interview transcripts indicate various transference phenomena, as well as identification mechanisms, that revealed the importance of the interviewers in some of the Bay Area women's (and sometimes their husbands') lives.

By "transference," psychiatrists and sociologists mean the ways in which interviewers come to "stand for" significant others or experiences in the lives of the people they are interviewing and thus generate feelings in the interviewee not directly related to themselves (Laslett and Rapoport 1975). For example: an interviewer asked Mary Yale to write (after her proposed move out of state), and "she says she'll try, but it's difficult to write letters now, even to her mother. I said, 'It wouldn't be like writing to your mother.' She said, 'no, it would be more like writing to my father' (said rather lightly)." Transference may also be expressed through delusional material involving the researcher:

Mrs. Quinn also told me about a number of strange ideas she had when she first went into the hospital, and she stated that I am the first person she has said this to. As one example, she mentioned the fact that the first time I took her out on the grounds she "associated me with" a psychiatrist she used to work with. She stated that I looked something like him. Apparently she had the idea I was the same person.

A more sociological version of this process, which I call identification (Warren and Mauldin 1980), involves the researcher "standing for" the generalized, rather than significant (parental, marital, or psychiatric-authoritative), others. Observers in mental hospitals or mental-health courts (Warren 1982) have observed that when they speak to patients,

patients respond with comments that express a mutual identification with the socially normal, thus at least momentarily allowing the patient to escape from the special category of the stigmatized. The appeal is to the generalized other or to social standards that are held in common and in equality with the interviewer.

Since the interviewers attempted to remain reasonably uninformative about their own private lives, attempts at identification remained at the superficial level encountered in brief visits to mental hospitals or courts: comments directed at the interviewer's clothing, hairstyle, or behavior in relation to the patient's own were the most common identification expressions. For example, Eve Low's interviewer noted, "En route to the receiving suite, I mentioned that I was late because I'd gotten myself locked out of my car. She said, 'Oh my, that sounds like something I'd be likely to do.'"

It seems plausible that the clinical drift of some of the interviews was due to the fact that the interviewers were associated with the mental hospital in the patient's mind. However, this seems to be less of a factor than the interviewee's situated desire for the expression of feeling, transference needs, and so on. For the wives, the experience of emotional trouble seemed to be the force behind their search for therapeutic assistance from the interviewer. When similar interactions occurred in the interviews with husbands, this too reflected situational emotions and needs:

Tim Quinn: He then proceeded to ask me what I thought about his wife's condition, how long I thought she would be there, and what I think about the prognosis. I told him I can't answer his questions because I just don't know. He then said that I must have an opinion. I told him all I can say is that patients vary considerably and I would have no way of predicting in his wife's case. After a little more pressure from Mr. Quinn I finally suggested to him that what he's really concerned about is whether she will get out of the hospital and give him further trouble—that he's afraid he may find himself in the same unpleasant situation. His response at first was to say that he hadn't thought about it that way, and then after a pause said I was probably right. There was another pause and then Mr. Quinn leaned forward intently and said something like, "I guess the fact is that I don't want her to get better. That's an awful way to feel, isn't it?" I shrugged my shoulders and said something to the effect that well, we can't always feel the way we would like to feel. He then said something like, "No, but that's immoral isn't it?" I again shrugged my shoulders and said something intended to be neutral, but which was probably more permissive of his feelings than otherwise.

The Bay Area interviewers had been instructed not to act as clinicians or to give the respondents advice (Sampson et al. 1964); thus the respondents' search for clinical communications and information from the interviewers was met with evasions. Mr. Quinn, for example, complained that when he asked the interviewer for ideas about his wife's prognosis, "all he wanted was an opinion. Instead of this I was evasive with him or stated that I couldn't tell him because this was something that was up the hospital. . . . He reminded me that he had told me during our first interview that this is a 'two way street.'" On occasion, the interviewers did provide the respondents with what they sought. Joyce Noon's interviewer admitted, "I had originally anticipated that I would stop the interview after about one tape, but since Joyce seemed to be getting some benefit from talking to me and expressing her feelings, I went on for another tape to give her further opportunity to do so."

Triadic Relationships

Some of the special shape of the interviews in this research came from the practice of assigning one interviewer to both spouses' interviews over time. Also, of course, the assigned interviewer was either a male or a female. The combination of gender, interviewing over time, and the conflicts in the typical Bay Area marital relationship produced some interesting triadic relationships within the research process.

Georg Simmel's analysis of triadic relations offers a number of insights for interpreting the problems reported by the Bay Area interviewers in their attempts to maintain interview contact with both husbands and wives, in separate and in joint interviews (1950). Simmel describes three contexts of triadic relations: the intimate, in which the dyadic marriage becomes a triad through childbirth; the situation of a subordinate and superior when a third element is added; and the social situation of the nonpartisan mediator or arbitrator who deals with dyadic conflict. The researcher who must interview both husbands and wives is to a degree in the situation of the nonpartisan, described as follows by Simmel: "The third element is non-partisan either if he stands above the contrasting interests and opinions (of the dyad) and is actually not concerned with them, or if he is equally concerned with them . . . the non-partisan may make the interaction between the parties and between himself and them, a means for his own purposes" (ibid., 149–150).

The researcher is in the position of the nonpartisan in the sense that he is (or rather his research task is) concerned equally with both. But in practice, there were frequent attempts on the part of one spouse to seek confidential information or to form a coalition with the researcher against the other:

Floyd Sand: Mr. Sand told me that he didn't see any point going on (with the interviews). . . . He asked me if I had talked to his wife that day and when I did not answer at once he repeated the question and I finally told him that I did. . . . He told me that this wasn't going to help him anyway, and besides which, I knew things about what was going on at the hospital with his wife, and I didn't tell him a thing about it. He brought this up a few times . . . saying that a person isn't much of a friend if he hides important things like this [his wife had been having an affair, which the interviewer did in fact know about] from someone. . . . [later] He . . . said with a smile that maybe he could subpoena me for [the court hearing on his wife's recommitment]. (I don't know if I looked sick, but I certainly felt it.) He went on in this vein, showing considerable glee, saying that being I knew both sides of the picture, that I could testify about them at the hearing. . . . During this talk with him I was debating, in my mind, whether or not I should tell him that his wife was being discharged from the hospital that day. I figured that he would find out about it eventually and that if I didn't tell him now this would aggravate this sore point about my keeping information from him. However, in view of the fact that he was obviously not expecting his wife out, and that the news of such was likely to provoke a strong reaction, and lead to some possible action on his part, I refrained from doing so. However, as I think about it, I do not believe that this will amount to too much, in terms of affecting chances for future contacts. I believe that if I continue to just drop in on him at his [place of work as a small-business owner], then there would be very little that he could do to avoid me, plus the additional fact that he would probably be under a lot of tension and feel the need to talk and present his side and gain a sympathetic ear, whatever his feelings about the use of all this.

Dyadic coalitions within the interviewer–wife–husband triad took several forms. Joan Baker continued to allow the interviewer to see her in the posthospital phase but kept the existence of these interviews secret from her estranged husband. She appeared to be afraid that if he knew she was still being interviewed by someone whom they both defined as associated with Napa, that meant she was still under psychiatric authority and thus still mentally ill. She told the interviewer, "I never told Arnold about you—I don't know why—except he has always said I had no business putting myself where I did. He said, 'since you did, just forget about it, don't let it bother you.'" The isolation of the housewife's existence ironically facilitated the maintenance of illicit relationships with either an interviewer or "the other man."

Sometimes it turned out that the marital partners had conspired together to keep information from the researcher that they knew would interest her or him. In the case of the Thornes this withholding took the form of a collusive withdrawal from the interview process. In other cases, the spouses had continued to involve themselves in the interview process, but were found at some later time to have deliberately misled or withheld information from the interviewer, generally because of fears connected with leave-of-absence rules and the authority of the mental-health system.

In joint interviews with the Bay Area spouses, the interviewer some-times took on the facilitating functions of the clinical–marital coun-selor: of a joint meeting with the Whites, the interviewer noted, "I would like to note . . . that several times during this interview both patient and husband remarked to each other to the effect that they hadn't realized the other had held the view just expressed." However—and as also in the clinical–marital counseling situation—the presence of the interviewer at times exacerbated some of the difficulties within the dyad, becoming, as Simmel calls him or her, a tertius gaudens (1950):

Whites (joint): The husband was in a way coaching his wife as to what to bring up for a discussion with me and as to what to say. He would frequently tell her, "Tell Dr. about such and such, or didn't you want to say something about this, or, was there a question you wanted to ask Dr." I could see some of the frustration that Mrs. White had in dealing with her husband . . . I also feel that part of Mrs. White's increasingly negative attitude toward psychiatry and thus I assume me, at this time, was fostered by the fact that her husband tried to move in the direction of some sort of alliance with me. At least he seemed to try to protect me at times from her more negative comments about psychology.

Even where jealousy was not a factor, the use of female interviewers with male respondents, and vice versa, precipitated some concern among the respondents about their perceived respectability in the neigh-borhood. This concern led to various modifications of the interview situation in the posthospital stage. Cora Thorne, for example, required the male interviewer to meet her at the laundromat rather than at home so that the neighbors wouldn't gossip. And when the male interviewer wanted to meet for coffee somewhere, she wondered "how it would look to the neighbors."

The interdependence of methods with situations and social structure is clear from these examples. The social place of the women respondents was within the traditional fifties family, as housewives and as mothers. Thus, the tasks they had to perform took precedence over the inter-viewer's agenda when they were at home and were irrelevant to it when they were in the mental hospital. The troubles that beset these respondents' unequal marriages were at the forefront of consciousness during the crisis phase of hospitalization, but such issues were deliberately banished from experience during the first days of return. From their different understandings of the world, the wives and husbands told the interviewer rather different tales. The husbands wanted company, attention, and a source of information during the wife's hospitalization; later, they wanted the ever-demanding interviewer to go away. And these are only a few examples. I would like to propose that such factors be taken into account when assessing the interview process, in contrast to the preference for focusing on the interviewer's establishment of rapport.

The Myth of Rapport

While participant-observational research relations have frequently been framed within the myth of trust (for a critique of this approach, see Warren 1983), the equivalent myth in intensive interviewing is that of rapport. By referring to these concerns as "mythic" I do not intend to dismiss them as of no importance in research relations. But it is important to realize that these concepts are used by researchers to gloss over complexities of communication between themselves and respondents and, in some cases, to deny respondents' experience of reality—precisely the opposite stance of that required by the interpretive method.

The concept of rapport implies that the interviewer can manipulate his or her own personality characteristics, and the interaction during the interview, to maximize respondent communication. Any breakdown in this process is viewed either as faulty method on the part of the interviewer or as denial (psychodynamically conceived) on the part of the respondent. Both approaches deny the respondent power to define or alter the situation.

The reality of the Bay Area women was centered, during the inpatient stage of the moral career, on hospital life, and during the ex-patient stage on housewifery and child care. Thus, a lack of smooth interaction during the interviews could be traced to the fifties housewife's social place during these different career stages rather than just to features of the interviewer's style and technique. Furthermore, such matters of setting may be everyday and not necessarily psychodynamic in character.

One consistent feature of the posthospital interviews—at least those that did not go smoothly—was that the interviewers attributed access and response problems to denial on the part of the respondent. A refusal to discuss the events of the previous stage, or a reluctance to continue the interviewing process, was seen as based on psychological mechanisms rather than everyday-life contingencies. The interviewees, however, framed their refusals in terms of the interviewers interrupting their daily routine. Mr. Yale, for example, was irritated at the arrival of the interviewer on one occasion and commented, "Tonight we needed some eggs, and we were going to go out to get them, but we remembered we had asked you . . . so we couldn't go." Similarly, a number of the women were less than welcoming to the interviewer and were willing to talk only if they continued their household chores; interviews were conducted, therefore, in laundromats, kitchens, and bathrooms, and while vacuuming, canning fruit, and painting the interior of the house.

A similarly psychodynamic interpretation was given to a second aspect of interviewee reluctance to continue the process: expressing irritation at constantly answering the same questions or dwelling on the same themes:

George Yale: The interviewer attributes the Yales' increasing reluctance to keep appointments to resistance, which he explores; Mr. Yale attributes it to having exhausted the topic, "going over and over the same thing." He wants to stop, but has a sense of obligation due to "help" from the interviewer during the "trouble."

June Mark (26th interview): In response to a question about her readmission to Napa "I don't know doctor, I mean, don't ask me—I don't know a darn thing."

(27th interview, question concerning ward life on her readmission) "It's just so boring, nothing ever happens—I don't know—nothing to talk about."

In both these examples, the respondents' boredom was ignored by the interviewers, attributed to denial. But boredom after the twenty-sixth interview is more than possible; respondent denial or faulty interviewer rapport were not life's major realities in the fifties household.

The concept of rapport does have some limited application to the interview situation. It is only common sense that the interviewer's style and personality should not "put off" the interviewee; if it does, only those interviewees most desperate to talk will be interested in doing so. And in addition it appears from the Bay Area transcripts that rapport (like trust) has some situational application, especially if it is seen as a form of transaction between the situation of the respondent at that moment in intersection with that of the interviewer. For example, during a series of interviews characterized in the main by the respondent's apathy and declared determination to "say nothing," the interviewer noted several exceptions:

June Mark: She expressed considerable interest in me today, and there is much to indicate not only positive transference but an identification with her [sic] . . . particularly her comment about similarities in our clothing and her interest in my activities when not seeing her.

For the first time she has directly spoken to me of these feelings [of self-doubts and fear of stigma] since I last saw her in the hospital; although it may indicate increased trust in the relationship with me, it may also indicate an exacerbation of her symptoms—a break in the effectiveness of her controls.

While the psychiatric interpretation of these positive indications would stress the return of mental-illness symptoms, and a sociological one would aver that "finally" trust had begun, a more respondent-centered interpretation would seek to discover Mrs. Mark's moods and needs in that particular interview. Although this was not done one can speculate: it is possible that she was experiencing renewed symptoms; it is also possible that she was lonely and wanted to talk to someone—that she had emotional but not necessarily pathological needs. From an examination of the Bay Area interview set as a whole, it is clear that the interviewer-based sociological hypothesis, that trust or rapport has finally begun and will now develop, is not an adequate model to describe the process of interviewing over time.

It is a truism in the social sciences—at least in interpretive work—that findings are never independent of the means used to produce them. Intensive interviewing is a special kind of method with particiular parameters, not reducible to an inferior (or for that matter superior) form of ethnography. Using the intensive interview will be a variable experience for the users of it, depending on their location in history and in culture—in time and space and in the web of social relationships.

Bibliography

Alexander, Franz G. and Sheldon T. Selesnick. 1966. *The History of Psychiatry*. New York: Mentor.

American Psychiatric Association. 1952. *Diagnostic and Statistical Manual of Mental Disorders*. 1st ed., Washington, D.C.: American Psychiatric Association.

————. 1980. *Diagnostic and Statistical Manual of Mental Disorders*. 3d ed., Washington, D.C.: American Psychiatric Association.

André, Rae. 1981. *Homemakers: The Forgotten Workers*. Chicago: University of Chicago Press.

Bardach, Eugene. 1972. *The Skill Factor in Politics: Repealing the Mental Commitment Laws in California*. Berkeley: University of California Press.

Barham, Peter. 1984. *Schizophrenia and Human Values*. Oxford: Basil Blackwell.

Bellah, Robert N., Richard Madsen, William L. Sullivan, Ann Swidler, and Steven M. Tipton. 1985. *Habits of the Heart: Individualism and Commitment in American Life*. New York: Harper & Row.

Berger, Peter and Hansfried Kellner. 1970. "Marriage and the Construction of Reality: An Exercise in the Microsociology of Knowledge." In *Recent Sociology*, ed. Hans Peter Drietzel, London: Macmillan, pp. 50–72.

Berger, Peter and Thomas J. Luckman. 1967. *The Social Construction of Reality: A Treatise in the Sociology of Knowledge*. New York: Doubleday.

Bernard, Jessie. 1972. *The Future of Marriage*. New York: World Press.

Bittner, Egon. 1973. "Objectivity and Realism in Sociology." In *Phenomenological Sociology: Issues and Applicaitons*, ed. George Psathas, New York: Wiley-Interscience, pp. 109–125.

Blumstein, Philip and Pepper Schwartz. 1983. *American Couples: Money, Work, Sex*. New York: William Morrow.

Bozarth, Ollie Mae. June 1976. "Shock: The Gentleman's Way to Beat Up a Woman." *Madness Network News*, p. 27.

Braginsky, Benjamin M., Dorothea D. Braginsky, and Kenneth Ring. 1969. *Methods of Madness: The Mental Hospital as a Last Resort*. New York: Holt, Rinehart & Winston.

Brown, Phil. 1985. *The Transfer of Care: Psychiatric Deinstitutionalization and Its Aftermath*. London: Routledge and Kegan Paul.

Cameron, Norman. 1943. "The Paranoid Pseudocommunity." *American Journal of Sociology* 46:33–38.

Cherlin, Andrew J. 1981. *Marriage, Divorce, Remarriage*. Cambridge, Mass.: Harvard University Press.

Chesler, Phyllis. 1972. *Women and Madness*. New York: Avon.

Chodorow, Nancy. 1978. *The Reproduction of Mothering: Psychoanalysis and the Sociology of Gender*. Berkeley: University of California Press.

Clausen, John A. and Marian R. Yarrow. November 1955. "Paths to the Mental Hospital." *Journal of Social Issues* 2:25–32.

Conrad, Peter and Joseph W. Schneider. 1980. *Deviance and Medicalization: From Badness to Sickness*. St. Louis: C. V. Mosby.

Corry, Barbara. November 1984. "Probation Officers' Techniques of Neutralization: Adolescent Rapists." Paper presented at the Annual Meeting of the American Society of Criminology, Cincinnati, Ohio.

Denzin, Norman K. September 1983. "A Note on Emotionality, Self and Interaction." *American Journal of Sociology* 89:402–409.

Diamond, Timothy. October 1983. "Nursing Homes as Trouble." *Urban Life* 12:269–286.

Dies, Robert R. April 1968. "Electroconvulsive Therapy: A Social Learning Interpretation." *Journal of Nervous and Mental Disorders* 146:335–336.

Easterlin, Richard A. 1968. *Population, Labor Force, & Long Swings in Economic Growth*. New York: Columbia University Press.

Elder, Glenn H. 1974. *Children of the Great Depression*. Chicago: University of Chicago Press.

Emerson, Robert M. 1981. "On Last Resorts." *American Journal of Sociology* 87:1–22.

——— and Sheldon L. Messinger. December 1977. "The Micro-Politics of Trouble." *Social Problems* 25:121–134.

——— and Melvin Pollner. December 1977. "Dirty Work Designations: Their Features and Consequences in a Psychiatric Setting." *Social Problems* 25:243–254.

Estroff, Sue E. 1981. *Making It Crazy: An Ethnography of Psychiatric Clients in an American Community*. Berkeley: University of California Press.

Ferraro, Kathleen J. October 1983. "Negotiating Trouble in a Battered Women's Shelter." *Urban Life* 12:287–306.

——— and John M. Johnson. February 1983. "How Women Experience Battering: The Process of Victimization." *Social Problems* 30:325–339.

Foucault, Michel. 1979. *Discipline and Punish: The Birth of the Prison*. New York: Vintage Books.

Frank, Leonard Roy, 1978. *The History of Shock Treatment*. San Francisco: self-published.

Friedberg, John. 1976. *Shock Treatment Is Not Good for Your Brain*. San Francisco: Glide Publications.

Glaser, Barney G. and Anselm L. Strauss. 1967. *The Discovery of Grounded Theory: Strategies for Qualitative Research*. Chicago: Aldine.

Goffman, Erving. 1961. *Asylums*. New York: Doubleday-Anchor.

———. 1971. "The Insanity of Place." In *Relations in Public: Microstudies of the Public Order*, New York: Basic Books, pp. 335–390.

———. 1963. *Stigma: Notes on the Management of Spoiled Identity*. Englewood Cliffs, N.J.: Prentice-Hall.

Gove, Walter R. 1975. "Labelling and Mental Illness: A Critique." In *The Labelling of Deviance: Evaluating a Perspective*, New York: Wiley, pp. 35–81.

——— and Jeanette F. Tudor. 1973. "Adult Sex Roles and Mental Illness." *American Journal of Sociology* 78:812–835.

Grosser, G. H. et al. 1975. "The Regulation of Electroconvulsive Treatment in Massachussetts: A Follow-up." *Massachussetts Journal of Mental Health* 5:12–25.

Gubrium, Jaber and David R. Buckholdt. 1977. *Toward Maturity: The Social Processing of Human Development.* San Francisco: Jossey-Bass.

Hartmann, Heidi L. Spring 1981. "The Family as the Locus of Gender, Class and Political Struggle: The Example of Housework." *Signs* 6: 366–394.

Hochschild, Arlie Russell. 1983. *The Managed Heart: Commercialization of Human Feeling.* Berkeley: University of California Press.

Holzman, Philips. 1977. "The Modesty of Nature: A Social Perspective on Schizophrenia." *Social Service Review,* 588–603.

Horwitz, Allan V. 1982a. "Sex Role Expectations, Power, and Psychological Distress." *Sex Roles* 8.6: 607–623.

———. 1982b. *The Social Control of Mental Illness.* New York: Academic Press.

Johnston, Roy and Karel Planansky. January 1968. "Schizophrenia in Men: The Impact on Their Wives." *Psychiatric Quarterly* 42: 146–155.

Katz, Jack. 1982. *Poor People's Lawyers in Transition.* New Brunswick, N.J.: Rutgers University Press.

Kolb, Lawrence C. 1973. *Modern Clinical Psychiatry.* Philadelphia: Saunders.

Laslett, Barbara and Rhona Rappoport. 1975. "Collaborative Interviewing and Interactive Research." *Journal of Marriage and the Family* 32: 968–977.

Laslett, Barbara and Carol A. B. Warren. October 1975. "Losing Weight: The Organizational Promotion of Behavior Change." *Social Problems* 23: 69–80.

Lemert, Edwin. 1962. "Paranoia and the Dynamics of Exclusion." *Sociometry* 25: 2–20.

Lidz, Charles W., Alan Meisel, Eviatar Zerubavel, Mary Carter, Regina M. Sestak, and Loren H. Roth. 1984. *Informed Consent: A Study of Decision-making in Psychiatry.* New York: Guilford Press.

Lofland, John and Lyn Lofland. 1984. *Analyzing Social Settings.* 2d ed., Belmont, Calif.: Wadsworth.

Lopata, Helena Z. 1971. *Occupation: Housewife.* London: Oxford University Press.

Lyman, Stanford M. and Marvin Scott. 1970. *Toward a Sociology of the Absurd.* New York: Appleton-Century-Crofts.

Lynd, Helen Merrill. 1958. *On Shame and the Search for Identity.* London: Routledge and Kegan Paul.

Maisel, Robert. Summer 1967. "The Ex-Mental Patient and Rehospitalization: Some Research Findings." *Social Problems* 15 : 18–24.

Margolis, Maxine L. 1984. *Mothers and Such: Views of American Women and How They Changed.* Berkeley: University of California Press.

Matthews, Jill Julius. 1984. *Good and Mad Women: The Historical Constructon of Femininity in Nineteenth Century Australia.* Sydney: Allen and Unwin.

McCarthy, Belinda Rogers. 1979. *Easy Time: Female Inmates on Temporary Release.* Lexington, Mass.: D. C. Heath.

Messinger, Sheldon L. Unpublished Bay Area study research notes, n.d.

———— and Carol A. B. Warren. 1984. "The Homosexual Self and the Organization of Experience: The Case of Kate White." In *The Existential Self in Society,* ed. J. Kotarba and A. Fontana, Chicago: University of Chicago Press.

Morse, Stephen J. 1984. *The Jurisprudence of Craziness.* Oxford: Oxford University Press.

Murphy, Jane M. March 1976. "Psychiatric Labeling in Cross-Cultural Perspective." *Science* 191 : 1019–1191.

Musgrove, Frank. 1977. *Margins of the Mind.* London: Methuen.

Oakley, Ann. 1974. *The Sociology of Housework.* New York: Pantheon.

Parsons, Talcott. 1951. *The Social System.* New York: Free Press.

Perruci, Robert. 1974. *Circle of Madness.* Englewood Cliffs, N.J.: Prentice-Hall.

Phillips, Derek L. 1963. "Rejection: A Possible Consequence of Seeking Help for Mental Disorders." *American Sociological Review* 28 : 963–972.

Physicians' Desk Reference. 1971. 25th ed., Oradell, N.J.: Medical Economics, Inc.

Pleck, Joseph H. 1985. *Working Wives/Working Husbands.* Beverly Hills, Calif.: Sage.

Pollner, Melvin and Robert M. Emerson. 1983. "The Dynamics of Inclusion and Distance in Fieldwork Relations." In *Contemporary Field Research,* ed. Robert M. Emerson, Boston: Little Brown.

Robitscher, Jonas. 1980. *The Powers of Psychiatry.* Boston: Houghton Mifflin.

Rokeach, Milton. 1964. *The Three Christs of Ypsilanti: A Psychological Study.* New York: Columbia University Press.

Rosenberg, Morris. September 1973. "A Symbolic Interactionist View of Psychosis." *Journal of Health and Social Behavior* 25 : 289–302.

Rosenhan, David L. 1973. "On Being Sane in Insane Places." *Science* 197 : 250–258.

Roth, Julius A. 1963. *Timetables: Structuring the Passage of Time in Hospital Treatment and Other Careers.* Indianapolis: Bobbs-Merrill.

Rothman, Michael Lewis and Robert P. Gandossy. October 1982. "Sad Tales: The Accounts of White Collar Defendants & the Decision to Sanction." *Pacific Sociological Review* 25 : 449–473.

Rubin, Lillian B. 1976. *Worlds of Pain: Life in the Working-Class Family.* New York: Basic Books.

Sampson, Harold, Sheldon L. Messinger, and Robert D. Towne. 1964. *Schizophrenic Women: Studies in Marital Crisis.* New York: Atherton Press.

Schatzman, Morton. 1975. "Paranoia or Persecution: The Case of Schreber." In *Labeling Madness,* ed. Thomas J. Scheff, Englewood Cliffs, N.J.: Prentice-Hall, pp. 90–119.

Scheff, Thomas J. 1966. *Being Mentally Ill: A Sociological Theory.* Chicago: Aldine.

———. 1975. "Labeling, Emotion, and Individual Change." In *Labeling Madness,* ed. Thomas J. Scheff, Englewood Cliffs, N.J.: Prentice-Hall, pp. 75–89.

Schur, Edwin M. 1984. *Labeling Women Deviant: Gender, Stigma, and Social Control.* New York: Random House.

Schwartz, Charlotte G. August 1957. "Perspectives on Deviance: Wives' Definitions of Their Husbands' Mental Illness." *Psychiatry* 20 : 275–291.

Scull, Andrew T. 1977. *Decarceration: Community and the Deviant—a Radical View*. Englewood Cliffs, N.J.: Prentice-Hall.

Sheehan, Susan. 1982. *Is There No Place on Earth for Me?* New York: Vintage Books.

Showalter, Elaine. 1965. *The Female Malady: Women, Madness, and English Culture, 1830–1980*. New York: Pantheon.

Simmel, Georg. 1950. *The Sociology*, trans. and ed. Kurt H. Wolff. New York: Free Press.

Smith, Dorothy E. January 1978. "'K is Mentally Ill': An Anatomy of a Factual Account." *Sociology* 12:23–53.

———. 1983. "No One Commits Suicide: Textual Analysis of Ideological Practices." *Human Studies* 6:309–359.

Smith, Kathleen, Muriel W. Pumphrey, and Julian C. Hall. 1963. "The 'Last Straw': The Decisive Incident Resulting in the Request for Hospitalization in 100 Schizophrenic Patients." *American Journal of Psychiatry* 120:228–233.

Stanton, A. and M. Schwartz. 1954. *The Mental Hospital*. New York: Basic Books.

Sykes, Gresham M. and David Matza. 1957. "Techniques of Neutralization: A Theory of Delinquency." *American Sociological Review* 22:664–670.

Szasz, Thomas. 1976. "Involuntary Psychiatry." *Cincinnati Law Review* 45:347–365.

Temerlin, Maurice K. 1968. "Suggestion Effects in Psychiatric Diagnoses." *Journal of Nervous and Mental Diseases* 147:349–358.

Thoits, Peggy A. September 1985. "Self-Labeling in Mental Illness: The Role of Emotional Deviance." *American Journal of Sociology* 91:221–249.

Warren, Carol A. B. 1974. *Identity and Community in the Gay World*. New York: Wiley-Interscience.

———. 1982. *The Court of Last Resort: Mental Illness and the Law*. Chicago: University of Chicago Press.

———. December 1983. "The Psychological Meaning of Mental Illness in the Family to Husbands and to Wives." *Journal of Family Issues* 4:533–558.

————. Spring 1984. "Toward a Cooptive Model of Qualitative Research." *Communication Quarterly* 32 : 104–112.

————. September, 1986. "The Mental Patient as Betrayer." *Journal of Health and Illness* 8 : 233–251.

————. 1987a. "Electroconvulsive Therapy, the Self and Family Relationships." In *Research in the Sociology of Health Care,* ed. Dorothy Wertz, vol. 8, Greenwich, Conn.: JAI Press, forthcoming.

————. 1987b. "Electroconvulsive Therapy: New Treatment of the 1980s." In *Research in Law, Deviance and Social Control,* ed. Andrew Scull and Stephen Spitzer, vol. 8, Greenwich, Conn.: JAI Press, forthcoming.

———— and John M. Johnson. 1972. "A Critique of Labeling Theory from the Phenomenological Perspective." In *Theoretical Perspectives on Deviance,* ed. Jack D. Douglas, New York: Basic Books.

———— and Linda Mauldin. Spring 1980. "Deliberation in Six Juries: A Participant–Observer Study." *Symbolic Interaction* 3 : 153–176.

Wells, D. A. July–August 1973. "Electroconvulsive Treatment for Schizophrenia: A Ten-Year Survey in a University Hospital Psychiatric Department." *Contemporary Psychiatry* 14 : 291–298.

Yarrow, Marian Radke, Charlotte Green Schwartz, Harriet S. Murphy, and Leslie Calhoun Deary. 1955. "The Psychological Meaning of Mental Illness in the Family." *Journal of Social Issues* 11 : 12–24.

Index

CPSIA information can be obtained
at www.ICGtesting.com
Printed in the USA
FSHW012144060122
87458FS